DR. C.

BSc., MPhil., BSc., PhD., CPsychol., AFBPsS.
Consultant Clinical Psychologist

The Technology of Diabetes Care

The Technology of Diabetes Care

Converging Medical and Psychosocial Perspectives

Edited by

Clare Bradley

Royal Holloway and Bedford New College, and
UMDS Guy's Campus, University of London

Philip Home

Freeman Hospital, and University of
Newcastle upon Tyne

and

Margaret Christie

Royal Holloway and Bedford New College
University of London

h● harwood academic publishers
ap chur • reading • paris • philadelphia • tokyo • melbourne

Harwood Academic Publishers

Post Office Box 90
Reading, Berkshire RG1 8JL
United Kingdom

3-14-9, Okubo
Shinjuku-ku, Tokyo 169
Japan

58, rue Lhomond
75005 Paris
France

Private Bag 8
Camberwell, Victoria 3124
Australia

5301 Tacony Street, Drawer 330
Philadelphia, Pennsylvania 19137
United States of America

Library of Congress Cataloging-in-Publication Data

The technology of diabetes care : converging medical and psychosocial
  perspectives / edited by Clare Bradley, Philip Home, and Margaret
  Christie.
     p. cm.
  Includes bibliographical references.
  Includes index.
  ISBN 3-7186-5084-3 (hard cover)
     1. Diabetes — Technological innovations — Evaluation. 2. Diabetes —
Psychological aspects. I. Bradley, Clare, 1952- . II. Home,
Philip. III. Christie, Margaret J.
     [DNLM: 1. Blood glucose —analysis. 2. Diabetes Mellitus-
psychology. 3. Diabetes Mellitus —therapy. 4. Insulin —
therapeutic use. 5. Technology, Medical. WK 815 7255]
  RC660.T43 1991
  616.4'6206 — dc20
  DNLM/DLC   91-7003
                                                                 CIP

Contents

Section 3: Technology in the Prevention and Treatment of Diabetes Complications

Section 4: Appropriate Use of New Technologies

Section 5: Evaluation of New Technologies

Preface

The development of appropriate technology, in medicine generally and in diabetes care in particular, is not a task for individual researchers but one for multidisciplinary teams. If we are to develop technology that will be effective in achieving the medical goal, whether it be lowering the blood glucose levels or reducing retinal complications, that technology must also be acceptable to patients and it must be usable within the constraints of the health care system and limited financial resources. Proper consideration of all these aspects of technology from the first stages of development will depend on active collaboration between researchers and clinicians from medicine and psychology, together with other health professionals and other social scientists where appropriate, and will always need to involve the active participation of the potential users of the technology, the patients themselves.

The purpose of this book is to encourage and facilitate multidisciplinary collaboration in the development of appropriate technology. The focus is on technology in diabetes care, although many of the issues addressed are equally relevant to the development of technology in other areas of medicine, particularly those areas concerned with the management of chronic illness. The book is written for researchers and clinicians involved in technology design and development and for those involved in the evaluation of technology in research studies or in clinical practice. Such researchers and clinicians might be medical doctors, nurses or other health professionals such as chiropodists or dieticians, or they might be psychologists, sociologists or economists. The book is written with all such readers in mind. A glossary of terms is provided to help promote effective communication across disciplinary boundaries and all authors have endeavoured to make their writing accessible to readers with diverse backgrounds. The book is suitable for teaching advanced undergraduate and postgraduate courses designed to educate and train researchers and clinicians who will be working at the interface of medicine with psychology, sociology, economics and other disciplines, such as ergonomics, which are concerned with the design, development and use of medical technology.

The book developed from a workshop on the technology of diabetes care held at the CIBA Foundation in December 1989. The workshop was organized by Clare Bradley and Margaret Christie of the Applied Psychology Research Group (APRG) at Royal Holloway and Bedford New College, University of London. The APRG's aim is to facilitate psychological research of relevance to problems and concerns outside of the psychological enclave. It holds regular working meetings and an annual workshop is held at the CIBA Foundation in London with contributions from a small invited group of participants. In 1989 the participants invited to the workshop included a wide range of health professionals involved in diabetes care, including a chiropodist, a diabetes specialist nurse and a general practitioner; hospital-based physicians and psychologists with special interests and wide-ranging experience in diabetes-related research; a sociologist and a health economist with experience in applying their disciplines to numerous areas of medicine; and representatives from both the British Diabetic Association and the World Health Organization. All of the speakers at the workshop and many of the other participants have contributed to this volume in which we develop further the work of the meeting at CIBA and communicate with a wider audience.

We would like to thank all the contributors for their efforts to meet the varied requests of the multidisciplinary editorial team together with the demands of new technology for 'disc manuscripts'. We thank the CIBA Foundation for their hospitality in providing us with their excellent facilities and the staff at CIBA, particularly Laura Shaw, Delia Betterson and Michele Canessa, for their warm welcome and efficient organization. We thank our generous sponsors, Novo Nordisk Pharmaceuticals Ltd, Ames Division of Bayer Diagnostics UK Ltd and Lilly Industries, for providing funds for the workshop and for their active interest in the proceedings and in the development of the book. Last but not least, we thank Amanda Sowden for her valuable assistance with the process of editing this book.

Clare Bradley
Philip Home
Margaret Christie

List of Contributors

HUW ALBAN DAVIES, Diabetic Unit, West Hill Hospital, Dartford, Kent DA1 2HF, UK

DAVID ARMSTRONG, Unit of Sociology as Applied to Medicine, Department of General Practice, Guy's Hospital Medical School, London Bridge, London SE1 9RT, UK

ALISON R. BISHOP, Diabetic Retinopathy Unit, Department of Medicine, Hammersmith Hospital, Du Cane Road, London W12 0NN, UK

CLARE BRADLEY, Applied Psychology Research Group, Department of Psychology, Royal Holloway and Bedford New College, Egham Hill, Egham, Surrey TW20 0EX, UK

JOHN BRAZIER, Department of Public Health Medicine, Medical School, Beech Hill Road, Sheffield S10 2RX, UK

CHRIS R. BREWIN, MRC Social and Community Psychiatry Unit, Institute of Psychiatry, De Crespigny Park, London SE5 8AF, UK

MARGARET CHRISTIE, Applied Psychology Research Group, Department of Psychology, Royal Holloway and Bedford New College, Egham Hill, Egham, Surrey TW20 0EX, UK

BRIAN M. FRIER, Department of Diabetes, The Royal Infirmary, Edinburgh EH3 9YW, UK

CHRIS R. GILLESPIE, Department of Clinical Psychology, Pastures Hospital, Mickleover, Derby DE3 5DQ, UK

DAVID A. HEPBURN, Department of Diabetes, The Royal Infirmary, Edinburgh EH3 9YW, UK

PHILIP HOME, Freeman Diabetes Unit, University of Newcastle upon Tyne, Newcastle upon Tyne NE7 7DN, UK

ALAN M. JACOBSON, Joslin Diabetes Center, One Joslin Place, Boston, MA 02215, USA

RICHARD JEAVONS, Northern General Hospital, Herries Road, Sheffield S5 7AU, UK

HARRY KEEN, Unit for Metabolic Medicine, Division of Medicine, Guy's Hospital, London Bridge, London SE1 9RT, UK

EVA M. KOHNER, Diabetic Retinopathy Unit, Department of Medicine, Royal Postgraduate Medical School, Du Cane Road, London W12 0NN, UK

JOHN R. KRAMER, University of Iowa Hospital, Iowa City, IA 52242, USA

THERESA M. MARTEAU, Unit of Psychology, Department of Psychiatry, Royal Free Hospital School of Medicine, London NW3 2QG, UK

KEITH A. MEADOWS, Department of Psychology, Royal Holloway and Bedford New College, Egham Hill, Egham, Surrey TW20 0EX, UK

WILLIAM D. MURPHY, University of Tennesee, 951 Court Avenue, Memphis, TN 38163, USA

JUDITH NORTH, British Diabetic Association, 10 Queen Anne Street, London W1M 0BD, UK

RICHARD B.S. NEWSOM, Diabetic Retinopathy Unit, Department of Medicine, Royal Postgraduate Medical School, Du Cane Road, London W12 0NN, UK

JOHN C. PICKUP, Division of Chemical Pathology, UMDS, Guy's Hospital Medical School, London Bridge, London SE1 9RT, UK

MASSIMO PORTA, Diabetic Retinopathy Unit, Department of Medicine, Royal Postgraduate Medical School, Du Cane Road, London W12 0NN, UK

CHRISTOPHER M. RYAN, 829 Savannah Avenue, Pittsburgh, PA 15221, USA

KIRSTEN STAEHR JOHANSEN, World Health Organization, 8 Scherfigsvej, DK - 2100, Copenhagen 0, Denmark

CHRISTOPHER STILES, Community Services Unit, Shaftesbury Road, Poole, Dorset BH15 2NT, UK

Medical and Psychosocial Perspectives on Diabetes-related Technology: Editorial Overview

Clare Bradley, Philip Home and Margaret J Christie

Joint appointment between Department of General Practice, UMDS, Guy's Campus, London Bridge, London SE1 9RT and Department of Psychology, Royal Holloway and Bedford New College, Egham Hill, Egham, Surrey TW20 0EX, UK.
Freeman Diabetes Unit, University of Newcastle upon Tyne NE7 7DN, UK.
Applied Psychology Research Group, Royal Holloway and Bedford New College, Egham Hill, Egham Surrey TW20 0EX, UK.

Evolution of Diabetes Care

Diabetes care is going through a period of rapid change, as indeed is the nature of patient care generally throughout other areas of medicine. The traditions of patriarchal medicine are loosening their hold with more collaborative approaches between doctor and patient taking over from the (usually) benign dictatorships of the past. Maybe these changes have been instigated by more enlightened practitioners, influenced perhaps by changes in medical education and increasing input from behavioural sciences. Maybe the changes reflect the changing demands and needs of patients with greater insistence from patients wanting to participate in decisions about their care, and greater levels of patient knowledge about the means and goals of diabetes management. Patients have always been concerned about the quality of their lives, levels of pain and discomfort, embarrassment, inconvenience and inflexibility of treatments. Patients are at least as concerned about the quality as they are about the quantity of their lives. However, clinicians have until recently failed to match their personal concern for the general well-being of individual patients with appropriate consideration and measurement of psychological, social and other variables outside the narrow band of medical variables which typically include only measures of metabolic control and of physical condition. The growth of a multifactorial perspective is reflected in contemporary psychosomatics (Christie and Mellett 1986), in behavioural medicine (Blanchard 1982) and in the massive development of health psychology (Stone 1990).

1

The Editors' Perspectives

The editors have each in their own way been aware of such changes. Philip Home as clinician and medical researcher has been at the interface between patients and technological developments. As editor of the journal of the British Diabetic Association, *Diabetic Medicine*, he has seen a steady increase in the number of papers submitted to the journal by psychologists and other social scientists and has played an important part in encouraging such submissions. The number of papers submitted by physicians using the tools developed by social scientists has also increased, together with the demand for reviewers who are social scientists involved in diabetes research. Margaret Christie as a psychophysiologist with close links with contemporary psychosomatics is very much aware of the need for greater interest in the interactions between biological, psychological and social factors; she has considerable experience of the problems arising when attempting to communicate across disciplines and specialties. Clare Bradley as a health psychologist has a major research interest in the applications of psychology to diabetes management. She has been involved with investigations of the role of psychological factors in several clinical trials of continuous subcutaneous insulin infusion pumps, including the World Health Organisation multi-centre European trial which is described by Kirsten Staehr Johansen in this book. She teaches health psychology both to psychologists and to general practitioners, and supervises many of their research projects, in her joint appointment between one of the medical schools (UMDS, Guy's campus) and a psychology department (RHBNC) at London University.

Technological Developments

In the first chapter Harry Keen outlines the technological developments considered in this book, ranging from developments in blood glucose monitoring technology, to glucose sensors and insulin delivery systems including insulin pumps and pen-injectors. Other technological developments, which hold at least as much promise for progress in diabetes care as those developments considered here, are beyond the scope of the present book. Notable among these are developments in information technology particularly developments in clinic record systems and developments in 'expert systems' to advise on diabetes management. Both of these developments in diabetes management have been pioneered by Peter Sönksen and his team at UMDS and St Thomas' Hospital. Other developments which are not directly considered here include transplantation of pancreatic islet cells, studies of the genetic components of diabetes, developments in drug technology aimed at preventing complications of diabetes and indeed at preventing the clinical manifestation of diabetes itself. However, although no chapters are specifically dedicated to these topics the issues considered here are highly relevant to all of these developments. Those involved in information technology developments at UMDS are more aware than most of the need for multidisciplinary collaboration between computer scientists, psychologists and physicians in developing and evaluating new information systems. The preferences and motivations, cognitions and emotions of patients and health professionals need to be considered in the development and evaluation of all technological developments. Consideration is given to the role of such psychological factors in the chapter by John Kramer and his colleagues and in the chapter by Clare Bradley within the section on evaluation of technologies. Also in that last section are chapters by Keith Meadows and by John Brazier and Richard Jeavons which give detailed consideration to the respective tasks of measuring quality of life and evaluation of economic factors. All of these issues are of central concern to researchers evaluating all forms of new technology in diabetes care and, indeed medical technology in general.

The Contributors' Perspectives

Several psychologists have contributed to the book: Keith Meadows with his background in psychometric design and development of diabetes-related measures has already been mentioned. Chris Gillespie is a practising clinical psychologist with clinical and research interests in diabetes management. John Kramer, Chris Ryan and William Murphy are psychologists who have been involved with the massive collaborative study of the effects of differing levels of metabolic control on development of complications of diabetes, the Diabetes Control and Complications Trial or DCCT. Here they collaborate with psychiatrist, Alan Jacobson, who has long standing involvement with diabetes research in general and the DCCT in particular, in writing about the psychological aspects of the DCCT. Chris Brewin, a research clinical psychologist, here in another multidisciplinary chapter, collaborates with Clare Bradley and Philip Home to apply a conceptual and methodological framework developed for assessing the needs of psychiatric patients to assessing the needs of people with diabetes. Theresa Marteau, a health psychologist, draws on her experience of the psychological impact of technology in many areas of medicine, including diabetes, in reviewing the literature and identifying pros and cons of technological interventions in diabetes care. Huw Alban Davis is both psychologist and physician who draws on both of these backgrounds in his research, developing computerised telemetric methods for use in management of diabetes during pregnancy.

Painting with a broader brush, David Armstrong, a medical sociologist who qualified in medicine before discovering sociology, provides a challenging view of the ways technology can be misused in attempts to manage people with diabetes instead of in management of the diabetes itself.

Physicians with a wide range of research interests in diverse technological developments have contributed to the book: all of these physicians are very much involved in diabetes care. As well as those mentioned above who have contributed to chapters first-authored by psychologists or who wear two hats themselves with their further qualifications in psychology or sociology, we have contributions from Harry Keen, professor of metabolic medicine at

UMDS, Guy's Campus, who has been at the forefront of so many developments in diabetes care and John Pickup from the chemical pathology department in the same medical school, well known for his work in developing and evaluating diabetes-related technologies. David Hepburn and Brian Frier write of their special research interest in insulin technology and the problem of hypoglycaemic unawareness that appears to be associated with certain insulins. Two groups of authors from Eva Kohner's Diabetic Retinopathy Unit at the Royal Postgraduate Medical School Hammersmith hospital have contributed chapters on the prevention and treatment of retinopathy. The groups include physicans Massimo Porta and Richard Newsom together with Alison Bishop, a diabetes specialist nurse colleague in the Unit. Kirsten Staehr Johansen from the World Health Organisation has a background as a dentist, a physician and as a clinical microbiologist and is now in charge of the WHO programme to promote quality assurance and appropriate use of medical technologies.

Contributing yet further perspectives to the book we have Judith North who wrote her chapter while heading the youth department of the British Diabetic Association and Chris Stiles, a chiropodist with a special interest in diabetes care who has been very aware of the importance of psychosocial factors in diabetes mangement and the untapped potential of the chiropodist for promoting whole person care. Last but not least we have the perspectives of health economists, John Brazier and Richard Jeavons. John Brazier writes from a Medical Care Research Unit while Richard Jeavons is Director of Resource Management in a hospital setting, with endless opportunity for involvement with difficult decisions about resource allocation!

Why Attempt to Facilitate Convergence of Perspectives?

Traditional medical perspectives continue to dominate some aspects of diabetes care, especially where technology is involved. Unless economic, psychological and sociological perspectives are also allowed to influence the design, development and evaluation of new technologies, those technologies will all too often turn out to be too expensive on resources, unacceptable to patients, damaging to patients' quality of life or destructive to relationships between health professionals and patients. With the help of psychosocial perspectives, health professionals can better look beyond assigning labels of 'non-compliant' to patients who do not follow their recommendations and instead of trying to fit the patient into the technology which the health professional believes is best, we should aim to design and use the technology in a manner which better suits the psychological as well as the medical needs of each individual patient. David Armstrong in his chapter on the social context of technology in diabetes care considers how technology has sometimes been used not so much to help control the diabetes as to control the person who has the diabetes. He suggests that one of the effects of this 'technology of control' is that patients are "reconstructed from the innocent victims of an unfortunate disease to the culpable and capricious agents of their own misfortunes" and that "the nature of the illness is changed in unintended ways, and with it the form of the interaction between doctor and patient".

Psychologists unfamiliar with the issues of diabetes and its management are often approached by diabetologists wishing to use the tools of psychology to research 'non-compliance' and establish 'what is wrong with' the IQ, personality, beliefs and cognitions of the patient who does not follow the doctor's advice. Such psychologists may unwittingly find themselves responding to and working within the assumptions of a medical perspective, unless they gain an understanding of the nature of diabetes and the available treatments and take a close look at the beliefs and behaviour of the health professionals as well as the patients. Shillitoe (1988) has provided an overview of psychology and diabetes which should prove valuable in informing health professionals unfamiliar with psychology as well as psychologists new to diabetes. Progress away from destructive views of 'non-compliance' will be made if such psychologists are able to communicate their own perspectives to their medical colleagues and those perspectives help to guide clinical decision making and formulation of research questions.

Physicians unfamiliar with psychology and its applications to diabetes care all too often shy away from the complexities and uncertainties of the people who have diabetes and express their concern for those people's condition by focusing on specific aspects of their metabolism or particular technological developments where the issues seem more straightforward. However there is a danger that the *individuals* with the diabetes are lost sight of, their psychology either ignored or assumed but not studied. The standard medical training does not normally equip medical researchers to tackle the complexities of research into human subjects; clinical and research collaboration with psychologists and other social scientists is one way towards overcoming some of the limitations of a medical training.

How Do We Attempt to Facilitate Convergence of Perspectives?

On 1st December 1989 Clare Bradley and Margaret Christie ran a workshop on the technology of diabetes care at the CIBA foundation in London. The workshop was one of a series organised by the Applied Psychology Research Group (APRG) at Royal Holloway and Bedford New College. The APRG is chaired by Margaret Christie and it was she who saw the potential of a workshop on technology and diabetes care and recruited the help of Clare Bradley to bring together the participants. All of the participants in the workshop have contributed to the book and Philip Home was, in addition to his contribution of a chapter on implantable insulin pumps, invited to join with Bradley and Christie in the editorial process. All chapters were reviewed by all the editors. We have all learnt a great deal in the process and we hope that the contributors and readers will too. The chapters vary widely in their perspectives of technology and their perspectives of patients. Although some convergence of perspectives was apparent during the workshop itself and even more apparent between first and final drafts of several of the chapters, the backgrounds of the authors clearly have a powerful influence on the different views of technology presented in their chapters. Where many of the technological developments described here are concerned, the meaning of the technology to the patient user has yet to be explored. Where this is the case authors can do no more than speculate and consider how psychological factors might influence the use of the technology. However, this in itself is valuable in identifying areas where research is needed. There is, for example, a need for research into patients' views of screening for retinopathy. We have come across patients who no longer believed themselves to be at risk of retinopathy because they had been screened. They had a notion that a negative result at one screening somehow guaranteed immunity from retinopathy. Other patients given the 'all clear' on screening, have taken this as the go ahead to continue with a low level of self care. How such misunderstandings can arise and how they can best be avoided are important questions amenable to research. Unless such research keeps pace with the technological developments the potential of those technological developments will not be realised and their value may be undermined. In the magnificent efforts to save eyesight with innovative technology it is easy to overlook the importance of just exactly what patients are told and led to understand, or have not been told and have come to believe about the screening process, and the effects such beliefs have on their behaviour.

Multidisciplinary collaboration requires great effort to appreciate different viewpoints, to communicate across the language and conceptual barriers and tolerate the frustrations that arise. The process of interdisciplinary collaboration is at times infuriating, perhaps because the superficial differences in language used so often represent just the tips of icebergs of different perspectives with different concepts and models of human behaviour. Nevertheless the outcome of multidisciplinary collaboration can be highly rewarding in terms of insights gained and progress made towards the appropriate use of technology in diabetes care. We appreciate the efforts made by authors who have responded so constructively to workshop participants' and editorial encouragement to consider alternative perspectives to their own, whether they be medical or psychosocial perspectives. We look forward to the continuing convergence of perspectives and future developments of ever more appropriate technologies in diabetes care.

The following two chapters by Harry Keen and by David Armstrong, set the scene for the book with two contrasting perspectives one from metabolic medicine and the other from medical sociology. Both authors are well known for their ability to cross disciplinary boundaries and report on what may be found in other territories.

References

Blanchard E.B. (1982) Behavioral medicine: past, present, and future. *Journal of Consulting and Clinical Psychology* **50** 795-796.

Christie, M.J. and Mellett, P.G.(eds) (1986) *The Psychosomatic Approach: contemporary practice of whole person care* John Wiley and Sons, Chichester

Shillitoe, R.W. (1988) *Psychology and Diabetes*. Chapman and Hall, London

Stone, G.C. (1990) An international review of the emergence and development of health psychology. *Psychology and Health* **4**, 3-1

Technology and the Diabetic Patient: An Overview

Harry Keen

Unit for Metabolic Medicine, UMDS, Guy's Campus, London Bridge, London SE1 9RT, UK.

Introduction

Young diabetic patients owe their lives to technology. After the first successful extraction of the hormone insulin from animal pancreas in 1921, its purification and its presentation in stable solutions of precise concentration were achieved over the course of an amazingly short time period. Within months the processes had been scaled up from the laboratory bench to the industrial production line and the life saving solution distributed all over the world (Bliss, 1982).

The Impact of Insulin

This behind the scenes industrial technology is usually far from the consciousness of the patient, but not so for those with diabetes. It made an impact very rapidly and directly upon the patient's life. Insulin must be administered by injection; injection requires syringe/needle assembly and skilled self-administration procedures for the patient to learn. A dose of insulin must be carefully measured; too much or too little may be dangerous, even devastating. The goal of diabetes treatment is to 'normalise' blood glucose concentration. In some way, then, glucose concentration must be measured, generating information which feeds back to regulate insulin dose and food intake. For decades, self-urine testing was the nearest the patient could get to estimating blood glucose. If blood glucose exceeded the 'renal threshold' (at about 10mmol/L or 180 mg/dl) then glucose would spill into the urine, its concentration there crudely reflecting the degree to which the renal threshold for glucose had been exceeded. If the urine was 'negative' the concentration of glucose in the blood could be anywhere from 10mmol/L down to zero! The correlation between glucose concentration in the urine and that in the blood was in any case of a very low order and sometimes downright misleading.

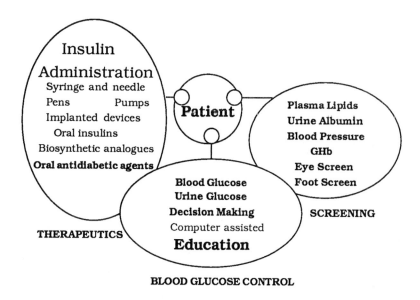

Figure 1. Three Main Areas of Impact of Diabetes Technology upon the Patient:

Therapeutics: The need to inject insulin has called for the development of specialised syringes and needles, portable insulin delivery pumps and multiple-charge insulin pens, easily carried by the patient. DNA technology scored its first major success in the biosynthetic production of 'human insulin', made by genetically programmed bacteria.

Blood glucose control: The response to insulin must be checked by monitoring blood glucose. This has become another major field of technical endeavour with the manufacture of specially prepared glucose sensitive strips and meters for reading strips. Decision making vis a vis insulin dose (or quantity or timing of food intake) can now be computer assisted with an algorithm to determine the dose and diet strategy.

Screening: Screening for early manifestations of diabetic complications has assumed great importance since effective preventive interventions have appeared. Visual inspection of the retina can be buttressed with retinal photography, recently with digitised laser imaging. Laser photocoagulation of the retina has been shown greatly to reduce the risk of diabetes-related blindness. Kidney disease can be detected by urinary albumin radioimmunoassay, arterial obstruction by doppler ultrasound velocity profiles. Foot ulceration can be prevented by pedobarometry. Blood pressure measurement with the clinical sphygmomanometer is probably the simplest but most beneficial piece of technology for the patient.

Blood Glucose Self Measurement

The development in the 1970's of self testing strips for measuring glucose directly in the blood was a diabetes management breakthrough of major proportions. With sound training, patients could now take much fuller command of their diabetic control, monitor and modify their own response to treatment (Scott and Tattersall, 1986). The technology of the strip was simple but ingenious. An enzyme impregnated into the active end of the strip liberates oxygen from glucose which combines with a colourless compound to give a blue colour. The more the glucose, the more the oxygen liberated and so the denser the blue colour. With careful handling of the strip, a reflectance meter can read the depth of colour and give glucose concentration estimates which correlate very closely with laboratory bench estimations.

Action from Information

Handed all of this information, what are patients to do with it? Do they want to do it in the first place? Many sick people would like to hand over their medical problem to the doctor, yet here is the doctor trying to hand it back to the patient! The crucial decision the patient has to make, once or several times a day, is how much insulin to inject: the usual, prearranged dose if the blood glucose is correct, rather more if it is too high, less if it is too low, modified perhaps if there is some anticipated change in mealtimes, meal size or physical exertion. These can be most difficult decisions to make, often generating anxiety about the consequences of an incorrect decision. Technology again can come to the rescue. A small computer accepts the blood glucose data. On the basis of an algorithm, perhaps developed from experience in the individual patient, it can suggest the correct insulin dose and even advise on when next to measure the blood glucose and what to do on the basis of the value found. Subsequent chapters by Armstrong, Gillespie, Alban Davis and Marteau explore these issues further.

Open and Closed Loops

The methods described above form an open loop system for feedback control of blood glucose. The patient measures the blood glucose, considers the value (or allows a computer to do so) then decides on that basis what dose of insulin to give. We are within sight of the next stage in technological development, the closed loop feedback system. In this an implanted sensor will continuously monitor blood glucose concentration, feeding the signal generated into a computer. On the basis of an individualised algorithm, the computer will regulate the output of an implanted inslulin pump which will in turn deliver the correct amount of insulin to return the blood glucose to normal. The chapter by Pickup in this book is concerned with the development of such glucose sensors.

Hypoglycaemia Technology

The diabetic state, characterised by greatly raised blood glucose is treated by measures to reduce that level to the normal range in order to avoid the immediate risk of diabetic ketoacidosis in insulin dependent patients and with a view to reducing the risks of long term complications in all forms of diabetes. In those making punctilious attempts to normalise there is an inevitable risk of 'overshoot', that is to say forcing the glucose concentration below the normal range. The effects of this 'hypoglycaemia' range from mild symptoms of sweating, shakiness, palpitations and slight confusion of mind on the one hand, to a deep, unrousable comatose state on the other. Hypoglycaemia is, not surprisingly, greatly feared by many patients; it may evolve very rapidly, sometimes with little warning. A device to detect and warn of oncoming hypoglycaemia before it embarrasses or disables the patient would be a technological boon. Hypoglycaemic sweating lowers the electrical resistance of the skin surface and devices sensitive to this characteristic have been developed to trigger an electric alarm. Unfortunately sweating from other causes may trigger the alarm incorrectly, while in some patients, confusion of mind may be well advanced before sweating occurs and triggers the alarm. An implantable needle sensor which actually measures glucose in tissues is now under development. It can be set to alarm when blood glucose is dropping below a critical level.

Pumps

Insulin injected two, three or more times daily only partially mimics the natural pattern of insulin delivery from the pancreas of the non-diabetic person. Continuous infusion of insulin under the skin from a small portable pump which can be boosted to meet the extra needs of mealtimes, gets closer to the normal insulin profile and this approach has been widely investigated since the first study was published (Pickup et al., 1978). While offering certain advantages in terms of improved diabetic control, the pump presents the user with a relatively complex piece of equipment, which needs to be worn continuously and which necessarily makes demands in upkeep and maintenance. There is also a clear interaction between the pump and the patient. Some patients welcome the sense of control over their disease that the pump gives them; others feel that they are 'slaves of the machine' – 'bionic man' as one remarked – or that it is a constant reminder of their diabetic state. The place of insulin pumps has not yet finally been settled though it seems an appropriate treatment modality for a relatively small segment of the insulin-dependent population (Knight *et al.*, 1984). The quite clear improvement in glycaemic control that it produces can be closely matched at less financial cost by intensified injection regimens with three or four injections a day (Marshall *et al.*, 1987). The development of the insulin pen injector has made this more feasible. The place of the pump with depend in large part on patient preferences but also on resources of money and skill.

Pen Injectors

Insulin pens contain enough insulin for three or four days use, are capable of injecting measured doses subcutaneously with great simplicity and when not in use can be capped and carried much like a fountain pen. Though technically fairly simple in design and structure they are by no means immune to mechanical failure. Newly diagnosed patients started on pen injections must also be instructed in the use of standard syringe and needle techniques and this skill regularly retaught. There is little doubt that the pen confers greater feedom on the frequent insulin injector, a truly user-friendly technical contribution (Jefferson *et al.*, 1985; Walters *et al.*, 1985 and the chapter by North in the present book).

Oral Insulin

The quest for an insulin preparation that can be taken by mouth has gone on for decades. As a peptide, ingested insulin is inactivated by intestinal enzymes before absorption. Methods of protecting the insulin molecule against these enzymes have been developed by modifying its molecular structure to resist digestion or enclosing it within a lipid envelope in which it is absorbed intact into the portal circulation. Entering the body in this way, the insulin is delivered first to the liver, as is insulin secreted physiologically by the pancreas. There are potential theoretical advantages for insulin to access the system via the liver rather than via the general circulation. There are also many practical difficulties which are currently under research attack. Absorption of the insulin dose through the bowel wall is unpredictable, and major variations of insulin entry would not assist in obtaining smooth blood glucose control. Dose levels are likely to be very high so that a cost factor may enter the equation.

Biosynthetic Insulin

One of the first triumphs of the new recombinant DNA technology has been the production of insulin by genetically programmed bacteria and yeasts (Home and Alberti, 1982). Previously obtained entirely by extraction from animal pancreas, the past ten years has seen a conversion to biosynthetic insulin which approaches 100%. Technically it is no more complicated to programme a micro-organism to synthesise human as any other animal insulin and there may be minor immunological advantages in treating humans with human insulin. It removes the need for a complex network of pancreas collection and makes the supply essentially infinite in size. This technology is also capable of producing 'designer' insulins with different or special properties, such as more rapid absorption or longer duration of action.

Oral Antidiabetic Agents

The majority of people diagnosed as having diabetes are not insulin-dependent; unlike the minority group of characteristically more youthful patients, their survival is not contingent upon daily insulin injections. A proportion of these non-insulin dependent diabetic patients can lower their blood glucose toward normal with the orally active drugs, the sulphonylureas and the biguanides. The former work by stimulating increased insulin release from the pancreas and later by improving the responsiveness of the body tissues to that insulin. The blood glucose lowering mechanism of the latter is independent of increased insulin release and acts by slowing of glucose absorption from the intestine and enhancement of its uptake from the blood by the tissues. Much biochemical ingenuity has been directed to improving potency and reducing side effects of these useful drugs. Other families of drugs acting at other points in the metabolic pathway of glucose production and utilisation by the body are in the experimental pipeline.

Glycosylated (Glycated) Haemoglobin (GHb) and other Glycated Proteins

Glucose is normally present as a fuel in the blood and tissue fluids. It also has the property of combining, ultimately irreversibly, with many proteins in the body. The structural alteration caused by the glycation process may alter the functional characteristics of the proteins involved. For example, glycation of lens crystallin protein may contribute to the lenticular opacities occurring in diabetes. Glycation of lipoproteins or of their membrane receptors may alter the kinetics of the corresponding lipids. In this way, glycation may contribute to the long-term complications of diabetes. The degree of glycation, a non-enzymatic process, is related directly to the average height of the blood glucose. This property has been put to practical use in the case of circulating haemoglobin (Hb). Once transformed, the glycated Hb remains in the circulation until the removal of the erythrocyte, after an average existence of about 100 days. Thus the proportion of Hb glycated at a particular moment in time is an integrated resultant of the average blood glucose concentration of the preceding three months. It can thus be used as a broad indicator of average 'diabetic control' (Peterson and Formby, 1986). There is a number of glycated adducts of Hb, the key one of which used as a control index is often known as HbA_{1c}. Plasma proteins with much shorter biological half-life, are also glycated and so can serve as a much shorter term index (2-3 weeks) of glycaemic control.

The Technology of Screening

A major problem which confronts the diabetic patient is the risk of developing the long-term complications of the disease. The evidence which suggests that chronically elevated blood glucose levels increase the risk of microvascular complications (Tchbroutsky, 1978) is a major motivating factor for doctors and patients to strive to improve and maintain blood glucose control at near-normal levels.

Diabetic Retinopathy

Microvascular complications may affect the capillary circulation of the retina, leading to haemorrhages, formation of new vessels and fibrous tissue, and ultimately if untreated to blindness (Kohner, 1980). Regular screening of the retina with the clinical opthalmoscope has been a central feature of good diabetes care. Alternative screening methods by retinal photography have grown in popularity. High quality colour photographs of the retina can be reviewed and treatment initiated if risk factors appear. A new screening approach is with the Scanning Laser Opthalmoscope which generates a digitised computer image and has the potential for more detailed and analytical treatment of the retinal appearances. Ideally undertaken before the patient has suffered any visual symptoms, effective therapy consists of coagulation of sometimes large areas of the retina by either an intense white xenon arc light beam or, now more commonly, by laser beam, transmitted to the retina through the clear media of the eye. (See chapter by Newsom and colleagues in this book).

Early Diagnosis of Diabetic Kidney Disease

The kidney is also vulnerable to diabetes with progressive loss of the fine filtration vessels of the renal glomerulus (Viberti and Wiseman, 1986). At a late stage, when renal failure is established, the condition is irreversible though its rate of deterioration may be slowed by careful treatment of the accompanying raised arterial blood pressure. Over the past decade it has been shown that the patient destined to develop diabetic renal failure can be picked up much earlier in the course of the disease and given treatment which may stop or reverse the process. They can be detected early by demonstrating small but significant increases of albumin in the urine. At present this requires screening timed urine samples with a sensitive radioimmunoassay technique for measuring albumin at or near the very low concentrations that apply in non-diabetic people. Ingenious techniques for super rapid assay using immunoprecipitation techniques have made this test available for 'bedside' use and for regular outpatient screening. It seems likely that by its use, the scourge of diabetic kidney failure will be much reduced.

Obstruction of blood flow through the arteries leads to impaired function and even the death of tissues they supply. In the leg, arterial obstruction, which may ultimately lead to gangrene, can be detected by skin temperature changes, by a fall in the oxygen tension in the skin of the leg, by the use of doppler ultrasound probes which respond to pulsatile flow and, for relatively precise diagnostic purposes, by the radiographic techniques of difital subtraction angiography. Interference with coronary artery flow can also be defined by X-ray coronary arteriography. The insertion and inflation of a tiny baloon at the site of arterial narrowing can sometimes effectively restore a threatened circulation, the technique of percutaneous balloon angioplasty.

Risk Factor Reduction

Further back in the development of arterial obstruction the process can be halted or slowed by reducing the levels of certain lipids in the blood, particularly the cholesterol-rich low density lipoprotein particles and, in diabetic individuals, the triglyceride-rich very low and intermediate density lipoprotein (Frick *et al.*, 1987). The concentration of these damaging lipoproteins can be simply measured in tiny quantities of blood plasma on an automated machine. If found to be abnormal, they are correctible with diet or with lipid-lowering drugs.

Measurement of arterial blood pressure, using the familiar mercury sphygmomanometer, is one of the oldest technologies regularly applied to the patient and remains of very great value. High blood pressure, if unrecognised and untreated, is a major contributor to heart and kidney disease and to stroke. Sophisticated devices worn by the patient for continuous measurement of blood pressure are now available though their clinical utility remains to be fully evaluated. Of particular value to the diabetic patient is the development of new drugs to lower the blood pressure, devoid of some of the unwanted side effects of earlier preparations which caused postural symptoms, bowel and bladder problems with erectile impotence in men and disturbing metabolic changes in the composition of blood, fats and aggravation of diabetes.

Summary and Conclusions

This brief survey of the technology of diabetes care has been less than complete but gives some indication of the network of technology that enmeshes the management and self management of the diabetic patient. The growing role of the personal computer in record, analysis and corrective action has only been touched upon and is sure to develop in extent and power.

At the heart of this complex is to be found the patient to whom the technology may be seen as a blessing to ease the burden of diabetes and its complications or as a threat, a monster to be served if disaster is to be fended off. It is clear that explanation and training, for patients and for those who care for them, is essential if the benefits of technology are to be fully realised.

References

Bliss, M. (1982). *The Discovery of Insulin* McLelland and Stewart, Toronto

Frick, M.H., Elo, O., Haapa, K., Heinonen, O.P., Heinsalmi, P., Helo, P. *et al.* (1987) Helsinki Heart Study: primary prevention trial with gemfibrozil in middle aged men with dyslipidemia: safety of treatment, changes in risk factors and incidence of coronary heart disease. *New England Journal of Medicine* **317**, 1237-1245

Home, P.D. and Alberti, K.G.M.M. (1982) Human insulin. In D.G. Johnston and K.G.M.M. Alberti (eds) *Clinics in Endocrinology and Metabolism* **11**, 453-484. Saunders, London.

Jefferson, I.G., Marteau, T.M., Smith, M.A. and Baum, J.D. (1985) A multiple injection regimen using an insulin injection pen and pre-filled cartridged soluble human insulin in adolescents with diabetes. *Diabetic Medicine* **2**, 493-495

Knight, G., Boulton, A.J.M., Drury, J., Gamsu, D.S., Moses, J.L., Bradley, C. *et al.* (1984) A feasibility study of the use of continuous subcutaneous insulin infusion in a diabetic clinic: patients' choice of treatment. *Diabetic Medicine* **1**, 267-272

Kohner, E.M., McLeod, D. and Marshall, J. (1982) Diabetic eye disease. In H. Keen and J. Jarrett (eds) *Complications of Diabetes* Second Edition, 19-108. Edward Arnold, London.

Lebovitz, H.E. (1985) Oral hypoglycaemic agents. In K.G.M.M. Alberti and L.P Krall (eds) *Diabetes Annual* **1**, 93-110. Elsevier Science, Amsterdam

Marshall, S.M., Home, P.D., Taylor, R. and Alberti, K.G.M.M. (1987). Continuous subcutaneous insulin infusion vs injection therapy: a randomised cross-over trial under usual diabetic clinic conditions. *Diabetic Medicine* **4**, 521-525

Peterson, C.M. and Formby, B. (1986) Glycosylated proteins. In K.G.M.M. Alberti and L.P Krall (eds) *Diabetes Annual* **2**, 137-155. Elsevier Science, Amsterdam

Scott, A. and Tattersall, R. (1986) Self monitoring of diabetes: urine testing revisited and self monitoring of blood glucose updated. In K.G.M.M. Alberti and L.P Krall (eds) *Diabetes Annual* **2**, 120-136. Elsevier Science, Amsterdam

Tchobroutsky, G. (1978) Relation of diabetic control to development of microvascular complications. *Diabetologia* **15**, 143-152

Viberti, G.C. and Wiseman, M.J. (1986) The kidney in diabetes: significance of early abnormalities. *Clinics in Endocrinology and Metabolism* **15**, 753-782

Walters, D.P., Smith, P.A., Marteau, T.M., Brimble, A. and Borthwick L.J. (1985) Experience with Novopen, an injection device using cartridged insulin, for diabetic patients. *Diabetic Medicine* **2**, 496-498

The Social Context of Technology in Diabetes Care: 'Compliance' and 'Control'

David Armstrong

Department of Public Health Medicine, UMDS, Guy's Hospital, London SE1 9RT, UK.

Introduction

The last decade has seen the continuing development of technological solutions to the clinical problem of diabetes. These have included more effective ways of delivering insulin and considerable improvements to the technology which allows blood glucose to be measured. Yet while the delivery of adequate amounts of insulin at the correct time is clearly a technical problem, the imperfections of current technology mean that the control of glucose and insulin levels in the diabetic patient's body involve the intervention of human behaviour. Thus, until the advent of the total technological fix, such as effective transplants of pancreatic tissue or a usable automatic and self-adjusting insulin pump, it is not a biological homeostatic mechanism which must respond to changes in glucose levels, but human beings. Therefore doctor and patient behaviour are an integral part of the technological process by which the deficiencies of diabetes are redressed.

The medical goal of the care of patients with insulin dependent diabetes is the control of glucose through the control of insulin and carbohydrate intake. However, as the main intermediary between the doctor and the blood glucose level is the patient, what has happened is that the strategy of control has become increasingly directed at the patient. Technology, therefore, from being focused on repairing impaired biological mechanisms, is redirected to maintaining and enhancing control over individual patients and their behaviours. The effects of this 'technology of control' are various: patients are reconstructed from the innocent victims of an unfortunate disease to the culpable and capricious agents of their own misfortunes, the nature of the illness is changed in unintended ways, and with it the form of the interaction between doctor and patient.

Systems of Surveillance and the 'Cheating' Patient

The introduction of methods of glucose monitoring and measurement of glycosylated haemoglobin have given diabetologists a series of techniques through which patients can be interrogated to see if they are lying or cheating. For example, in 1984, Mazze and his colleagues provided 19 patients with glucometers which had been secretly modified to contain a memory chip. This meant that every time the patient monitored their own glucose with the glucometer and entered the result in a log book (at the doctor's request) the 'real' result was stored in the meter. Later, again unknown to the patient, the researchers were able to compare the stored results with those in the log book and find that "the majority of subjects displayed some degree of discordance between blood glucose levels reported in the logbooks and memory reflectance meter-recorded values" (p. 216).

The researchers were careful in their description of patients in the study – they were 'unreliable' or 'inaccurate' – and there were no recriminations for individual patients as the results were not revealed to them. However, although this group of 19 patients escaped being confronted with the discrepancies, the implications for others was more pointed. The research raised many questions, wrote Mazze and his colleagues, about "our ability to distinguish between fabrication, error, and accuracy": in short, could patients be trusted?

Other researchers joined the investigative thrust to identify just how much and how often patients did not speak the same truth as the machine with which they were secretly tagged. Hoskins et al (1988) carried out a similar study to that of Mazze and his colleagues to "verify the validity of glucose records" produced by patients' own self-monitoring – or, rather, to prove again the patient dissimulated. Again they found not only inaccurate readings but also those "results omitted and those invented".

Williams et al (1988) also gave glucose reflectance meters to patients who again "were not informed of the memory modules inside the meters". "Patterns of unreliable reporting" were discovered with 52% of patients showing discrepancy rates between logbook and meter-held values of at least 1 in 5.

In a further replication, Ziegler et al (1989) examined the 'reliability' of self-monitoring of blood glucose by using glucometers. Again, the meters had a memory capacity of which patients were unaware which allowed "discrepancies" to be identified. The authors claimed that the "aim of the study was not to pass judgement on the behaviour of patients ..." but there is little doubt that the technology offered its own assessment: if the technical apparatus spoke the truth then what were the patient's recordings?

The point of these studies is clearly to measure and refine the extent of patient 'dissimulation', but for what purpose? The repeated application of the same experimental design together with the same findings leads to the conclusion that the diabetologists should have a high level of suspicion about the degree of control that patients report. In an important sense, developments in the technology of control have simply revealed the lack of control which doctors formerly thought that they exerted: and the result is suspicion, frustration (Heszen-Klemens, 1987) – and another study to confirm that it really is true.

The suspicion of patients' veracity which the above studies engender has been further facilitated by another technological development in patient control, namely the measurement of glycosylated haemoglobin. Various studies have indicated a correlation between blood glucose levels over a period of several weeks and the level of HbA1. On the one hand this is a valuable tool in diabetes control assessment but in practice, like the reflectance glucometer, it has also been converted into an attempt to control the patient. Thus the level of glycosylated haemoglobin can be used to challenge the patient's own reports of control. From observations of doctor-patient encounters in diabetic clinics, Silverman (1987) noted the "moral framework" which this technique produced. This framework makes the consultation into a kind of trial for the patient in which he or she is held to be accountable for their actions. The power of glycosylated haemoglobin is "the ability to 'see through' patients' behaviour and dispense praise or blame" (p. 215). While directly charging the patient with lying was rare, Silverman (1987) found that in many consultations the doctor's (usually secret) knowledge that glucose control was not optimal was used to challenge patients' own claims to success, frequently in the form of getting patients to 'confess' their inadequacies or failings.

Limits of Technological Truth

Technological development in the care of diabetes may or may not have had an effect on the quality of care received by people with diabetes, but it certainly has had a very real impact in terms of constructing an 'unreliable' or even 'lying' patient. In effect the technology has had important unintended consequences which have served neither the patient's, nor in the final analysis, the doctor's own interests. Diabetologists have become caught in a web of technology which defines its own truth and ignores or represses any non-biochemical alternative view.

All the effects of new technologies need to be viewed critically. Technology does not function in a vacuum, independent of human actors; it is always *applied* to problems by people. The evaluation of the technology therefore requires the total process to be assessed, which includes the human intermediary. Thus rather than saying that reflectance glucometers give a true reading and that patients corrupt this truth, it is more correct to say that the *application* of such meters has only been of limited value in establishing blood glucose levels. In other words, it is the technology that has not worked. Indeed, rather than see a discrepancy between glucometer and patient's report as an instance of the patient 'lying', it is equally possible to explore the mismatch as revealing some truth about the way the patient is coping with the illness. Thus the technology speaks one truth (about the patient's biochemistry) and the patient speaks another about his or her experience of the illness.

Of course the mechanisms within the technological process can be further investigated to find out why it is of limited effectiveness. First, is the 'technical' component of the technology accurate? The assumption in the above studies was that the technical could not be the source of error in disagreement between the illness 'constructed' by the patient and the 'truth' revealed by the glucometer or glycosylated haemoglobin. But there are reports that glucometers can be inaccurate (Bradley and Moses, 1986). Even health professionals using the equipment have been found to produce discrepant results: Laus and his colleagues (1984) cautioned health professionals to be aware of the 'interdevice and intradevice variability'. And the 'truth', as revealed by glycosylated haemoglobin, is simply an indicator of underlying blood glucose levels with scope for individual variation. As Svendson and his colleagues have noted, "a given concentration of glycosylated haemoglobin may result from varying degrees of glucose control" such that "the usefulness of glycosylated haemoglobin determination in the assessment of long-term glycaemic control in the *individual* patient (is) rather doubtful" (Svendson et al, 1982: p.403).

Second, the behaviour of patients in the use of new technology can be explored – but not by studies which simply treat them as part of a machine and show their incompetence. The question is *why* patients play an active part in constructing their own biological parameters, and this can only be answered by asking them.

Social scientists have been interested in the behaviour of people with illnesses for the last 30 years. Initially, this interest focused on the failure of patients to take their illnesses to the doctor or to attend for screening and preventive activities. This emphasis on what became known as illness and/or health behaviour, tended to see the problem as simply one of information (Mechanic, 1962). If patients were aware of the implications of their symptoms, or the risks they ran in not having adequate preventive or screening activities, then they would not act in a medically irrational way. Hence the emphasis was on educating patients to behave according to medical rationality and expectations.

Social scientists' understanding of this problem became more sophisticated about a decade ago when it was noted that the "natural state" was not one of medical logic. Rather, medical rationality was simply one way of looking at the world, neither necessarily more coherent nor effective. This view emerged particularly from medical anthropologists who, in examining pre-industrial societies, discovered their members to have complex sets of explanatory models or lay theories for the various illnesses they experienced. This perspective was then applied to Western societies, and the discovery was made that members of these communities also had complex views about the nature of illness. Research showed that patients had views about the cause, effects, and appropriate treatment for various illnesses which were embedded in a wider context of explanation. Most patients seemed anxious to answer the questions: why me? why now? why this (particular disease)? (Kleinman et al, 1978). Very often, medical science could not answer these questions, and patients were left to supply their own answers from their own cognitive resources (Locker, 1981). For example, where diabetes is concerned, although doctors may have elaborate explanations for many of the biochemical processes involved, medicine is remarkably deficient in offering an explanation to patients about why *they* have got the disease, why it happened exactly when it did, and why they have got this disease and not another chronic illness.

Thus, within the context of these explanatory models which patients use to explain their illness, the role and meaning of technology has a particular place. As Kelleher observed in his book on the experience of diabetes (1988), the experience of the illness is in large part the experience of the technological control systems, rather than the disease. Thus the engagement of the patient's cognitive systems with the technology is as important as with the illness itself.

Technology as Mediating between Doctor and Patient

There are many different characterisations of the relationship between doctor and patient in the sociological literature. Broadly, these range from a view of common interest and consensus to different agendas and potential conflict (Armstrong, 1989). In most of these models both doctor and patient have resources at their disposal to promote their own agendas. However, in diabetes the available technology has enabled shifts in the balance of power between doctor and patient to come about. The advent of HbA1 screening in diabetes has enabled the doctor to "spy" on the patient and at times uncover lying. Patients have responded with strategies to try and overcome this technological imperialism, which threatens to reduce them to non-people, by constructing a blood glucose record which will please the diabetologist (Silverman, 1987). Fixing the biochemical record, however, is only one part of the extensive 'cognitive work' which patients with diabetes may engage in so as to cope with the meaning that the disease and its management holds for them.

Aside from the moral and ethical issues involved in attempting to evaluate patients' truthfulness and compliance, the effect of technology on the doctor/patient relationship might lead one to suspect that the nature of the relationship was being changed for the worse. In effect, the quality of the relationship, between a doctor potentially concerned about the whole illness and the patient who experiences it, can be usurped by the demands of the technology that patients should always speak the medical truth.

In this sense the use of new technology in the care of diabetes can both redirect the attention of the physician to controlling the patient rather than controlling the diabetes, and at the same time, transform the nature of the relationship itself.

Summary and Conclusions

As described in the introduction the advent of a technological fix which worked completely would transform the field of diabetes and make redundant any of the social issues raised above. But, in the absence of that perfect technological apparatus, it would seem that the behaviour of both doctors and patients have a major role to play in the application of technology to diabetic care. In fact, as this paper has argued, human behaviour becomes a part of the technology and is subsumed under it. Systems of control which had originally been directed at a biochemical process become, step by step, redirected towards a new objective, namely the control of patients themselves.

While not wishing to detract from the importance and the need to try and achieve a technological solution to the problem of diabetes, the above arguments would suggest that technology needs to be seen in its proper social context. Technology, from being a vital component of the solution to diabetes, becomes an important part of the problem. Just as diabetes is not simply a biological malfunction, in that it has psycho-social consequences and experiences for the individual patient, so, too, technology is not a neutral strategy: it has major effects on the beliefs and behaviours of both doctors and patients, which need to be taken into account in any assessment and promotion of further technological intervention. Far from treating patient's beliefs and behaviours as impediments to the proper functioning of professional diabetes care, it is time to recognise that these are both integral parts of the whole patient and, evidence is beginning to suggest, important components of successful management (eg. Bradley et al, 1987).

Acknowledgements

I am grateful to Clare Bradley for helpful comments on ealier drafts of this chapter.

References

Armstrong, D. (1989) *An outline of sociology as applied to medicine*. John Wright, London. 3rd edition.

Bradley, C. and Moses, JL. (1986) Evaluation of blood glucose measurement techniques: locating sources of error. *Diabetes Research* 3, 53–58.

Bradley, C. Gamsu, DS. Moses, JL. Knight, G. Boulton, AJM. Drury, J. and Ward, JD. (1987) The use of diabetes-specific perceived control and health belief measures to predict treatment choice and efficacy in a feasibility study of continuous subcutaneous insulin infusion pumps. *Psychology and health* 1, 133–146.

Heszen-Klemens, I. (1987) Patients' non-compliance and how doctors manage this. *Social Science and Medicine* 24, 409–416.

Hoskins, PL. Alford, JB. Handelsman, DJ. Yue, DK. and Turtle, JR. (1988) Comparison of different models of diabetic care on compliance with self-monitoring of blood glucose by memory glucometer. *Diabetes Care* 11, 719–724.

Kelleher, D. (1988) *Diabetes: the experience of illness*. London, Routledge.

Kleinman, A. Eisenberg, L. and Good, B. (1978) Culture, illness and cure. *Annals of Internal Medicine* **88**, 251–259.

Laus, VG. Dietz, MA. and Levy, RP. (1984) Potential pitfalls in the use of Glucoscan and Glucoscan II meters for self-monitoring of blood glucose. *Diabetes Care* **7**, 590–4.

Locker, D. (1981) *Symptoms and illness: the cognitive organisation of disorder.* Tavistock, London.

Mazze, RS. Shamoon, H. Pasmantier, R. Lucido, D. Hartmann, K. Kuykendall, V. and Loptatin, W. (1984) Reliability of blood glucose monitoring by patients with diabetes mellitus. *American Journal of Medicine* **77**, 211–217.

Mechanic, D. (1962) The concept of illness behaviour. *Journal of Chronic Diseases* **15**, 189–194.

Silverman, D. (1987) *Communication and medical practice: social relations in the clinic*. Sage, London.

Svendson, PA. Lauritzen, T. Soegaard, U. and Nerup, J. (1982) Glycosylated haemoglobin and steady mean blood glucose concentration in Type 1 (insulin-dependent) diabetes. *Diabetologia* **23**, 403–405.

Williams, CD. Scobie, IN. Till, S. Crane, R. Lowy, C. and Sonksen, PH. (1988) Use of memory meters to measure reliability of self blood glucose monitoring. *Diabetic Medicine* **5**, 459–462.

Ziegler, O. Kolopp, M. Got, I. Genton, P. Debry, G. and Drouin, P. (1989) Reliability of self-monitoring of blood glucose by CSII-treated patients with Type 1 diabetes. *Diabetes Care* **12**, 184–188.

B

1

BLOOD GLUCOSE MONITORING

In the previous chapter, David Armstrong considered how health professionals can misuse blood glucose monitoring technology in attempts to control the patients' behaviour rather than the diabetes in a manner which is likely to be destructive both in terms of diabetes control and staff-patient relationships. In the present section, the focus is on how blood glucose monitoring technology may be further developed and on constructive ways of using existing blood glucose monitoring technology with a view to improving collaboration between health professionals and their patients, and improving patients' blood glucose control while enhancing their quality of life.

In the first chapter John Pickup describes the promising new developments in glucose sensor technology. Development has been a long, slow process, with scientific, technical and psychological hindrances still to be overcome and the problems of communicating across the disciplines of engineering and medicine to be solved. Now the first of the glucose sensors are reaching the point where their potential uses can be evaluated. In the final section of this book, Clare Bradley uses the example of glucose sensors in considering how psychological factors can best be taken into account in evaluating new technologies in diabetes care.

Chris Gillespie reviews the literature on self monitoring of blood glucose (SMBG) including studies of ways in which SMBG might most effectively be used to improve metabolic control with the minimum of negative consequences. Initial assumptions that frequent, accurate measurement of blood glucose would somehow lead to improved glucose control have proved to be over optimistic. Patients must make active and appropriate use of the SMBG data if SMBG is to lead to improved blood glucose control.

One interesting development which is reviewed by Gillespie is the use of feedback from SMBG to train awareness of blood glucose. Those patients who are able to acquire reliable awareness of their blood glucose levels would effectively be able to monitor their blood glucose levels continuously. Here we see a psychological approach to a problem similar to that which glucose sensors are being developed to solve. Glucose sensors would be most useful to those patients unable to acquire blood glucose discrimination skills and those who were troubled by night time episodes of hypoglyaemia. Research has yet to establish the limits of blood glucose awareness training and to find ways of identifying which patients are most likely to benefit from the different methods of blood glucose monitoring that are becoming available.

In the final chapter in this section Huw Alban Davies describes one way in which SMBG data, recorded in the memory of a meter used by the patient, may be transmitted over the telephone for perusal by the hospital doctor, who may then hold a telephone consultation with the patient. The study described by Alban Davies involved pregnant women with diabetes, a condition in which optimal blood glucose control is known to be of great significance to the well-being of the developing baby. This model of collaborative care is in stark contrast to the adversarial relationships between doctor and patient implied in research studies using meters with hidden memories of which the patients are unaware in order to check up on the accuracy with which patients reported their meter readings. Collaborative relationships between doctor and patient are likely to be the most appropriate relationships for all people with diabetes, pregnant or not.

The uses to which blood glucose monitoring technologies can be put are many and varied. If the potential of such technologies is be fully realised the importance of psychosocial issues needs to be recognised. Evaluative research needs to focus not just on the techology per se but on the use to which the technology is put, if we are to avoid blaming the technology when it has been used inappropriately and if we are to demonstrate opportunities for its more appropriate use. Issues of evaluation are considered in detail in section 6.

Glucose Sensors

John Pickup

Division of Chemical Pathology, United Medical and Dental Schools, London SE1 9RT, UK.

The General Principles of Biosensor Operation

Glucose sensors belong to a class of measuring devices called 'biosensors' (Pickup, 1985). These are miniature probes or transducers where a biological receptor is attached to a detector so that a specific and rapid signal occurs when a chemical (analyte) binds to the probe. Biosensors are receiving considerable attention in many fields of clinical medicine and other areas (Turner *et al.*, 1987) because, potentially, they offer a number of advantages over many conventional measuring procedures which are currently used in laboratories and hospitals (Table 1).

Although many receptors have been employed in biosensors for measuring different analytes, including antibodies ('immunosensors'), whole cells, bacteria and tissue slices, most interest has been focused on enzyme electrodes, where the enzyme-catalysed reaction produces a change in potential, current, heat or light which can be detected by an underlying electrode (for potential and current), thermistor (for heat) or fibre optic (for light). Field-effect transistors are a special kind of microprocessor-based device for voltage measurements.

Table 1

Advantages of Biosensors (Such as a Glucose Sensor) Compared to Conventional Measurements

Can be miniaturised
Simple to operate
Reagentless
Will operate in turbid or coloured solutions
Do not consume or withdraw body fluid
May be mass-produced
May be operated continuously

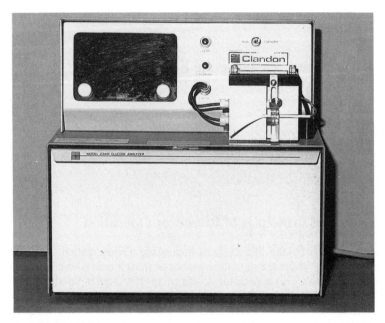

Figure 1. The YSI model 23, an example of a glucose sensor incorporated in a bench-top analyser for measurement of whole blood or plasma glucose concentrations. The dimensions of the analyser are 32 x 21 x 31 cm.

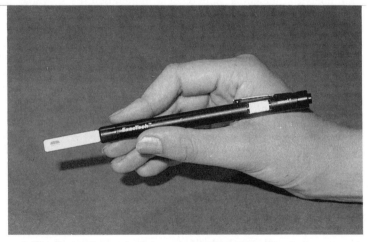

Figure 2. The Exactech pen. A glucose sensor for capillary blood glucose monitoring by patients. Blood is placed on the end of the strip which contains immobilised glucose oxidase and ferrocene on one pad and a silver/silver chloride reference at the other.

The Reasons for Developing Glucose Sensors

Like many sensors, glucose transducers can be used either *in vitro* in samples of body fluid such as blood or *in vivo* as an implantable device. *In vitro* glucose sensors perform discrete analyses and might therefore be useful for capillary blood glucose self-monitoring in diabetic patients or to produce smaller, cheaper or more efficient laboratory analysers. Fig. 1 shows a bench-top laboratory blood glucose analyser in current use (the Yellow Springs analyser) which is based on a glucose-sensing membrane, and Fig. 2 shows the recently-introduced pen-sized glucose meter (Exactech) for capillary blood measurement. Implantable glucose sensors naturally bring to mind the goal of constructing a closed-loop (feedback-controlled) insulin delivery system, a wearable artificial pancreas (Fig. 3a, 3b), but there are several other configurations which technically are more feasible in the near future and which are of at least equal clinical priority. One such is a hypoglycaemia alarm (Fig. 3d).

Figure 3. Diagrams to represent possible configurations of glucose sensors.

(a) Feedback-controlled insulin delivery ('closed-loop') where blood is pumped from a peripheral vein to a glucose sensor and insulin infused intravenously.

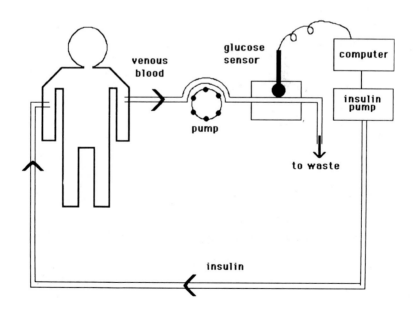

(b) A closed-loop insulin delivery system with the sensor implanted in the subcutaneous tissue and insulin infusion also into the subcutaneous tissue.

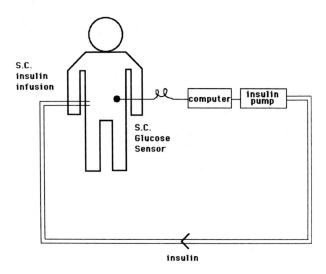

(c) An 'open-loop' system with direct read-out of glucose levels from a subcutaneously-implanted sensor.

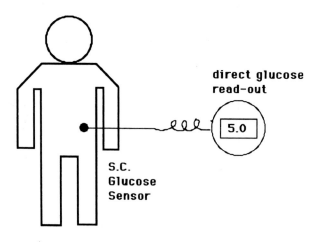

(d) A hypoglycaemia alarm based on a subcutaneously-implanted sensor.

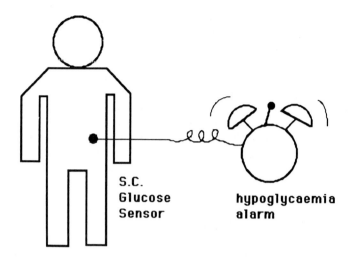

S.C.
Glucose   hypoglycaemia
Sensor   alarm

Hypoglycaemia is a common, potentially-hazardous and much-feared complication of insulin treatment. A hypoglycaemia alarm which could be activated at a preset glucose level and operated over just an 8–12 hour period (say overnight) would be both clinically very valuable and compatible with present achievements in sensor stability during continuous measurement. Hypoglycaemia detection would be particularly useful for those patients who have lost the warning symptoms of low blood glucose concentrations (Heller *et al.*, 1987).

A continuous or on-demand read-out of glucose levels *in vivo* (Fig. 3c) would clearly also aid insulin dosage adjustments and warn against dangerous hyperglycaemia and indicate the need for ketone body testing. Short-term continuous blood glucose sensing may be of value in diabetic patients at operation or during intensive care and, for this period of time, blood could be passed into a flow-through cell where glucose levels may be measured *ex vivo* (Fig. 3e). Although blood is not consumed by the sensor and theoretically could be reinfused into patients, the possibility of clot formation and/or the introduction of infection in *ex vivo* systems, argues that blood 'downstream' of the sensor should most safely be allowed to go to waste.

Glucose Sensor Technology

Glucose sensor research has been active for more than 25 years (Clark and Lyons, 1962). Most interest has centred on amperometric (current-measuring) enzyme electrodes based on monitoring oxygen consumption (Updike and Hicks, 1967; Gough *et al.*, 1985) or hydrogen peroxide production (Clark and Duggan, 1982; Shichiri *et al.*, 1982) at a platinum base electrode, with catalysis by immobilised glucose oxidase. Potentiometric (voltage-measuring) enzyme electrodes have also been employed where changes in (H^+) or other ion concentrations cause Nernstian voltage alterations (Caras *et al.*, 1985). Apart from insensitivity (potential varies with the logarithm of the analyte activity), potentiometric glucose sensors often suffer from varying response slopes. Electrocatalytic sensors which oxidise glucose at a noble metal catalyst without enzyme are a further alternative but they are prone to non-specificity and fouling, though more sophisticated wave forms of applied potential and signal analysis may overcome some of these problems (Lerner *et al.*, 1984). Optical approaches are at an early stage of development.

In spite of the long history of research and development in this area, it is only in the last two years or so (Matthews *et al.*. 1987) that a small, probe-type device which could genuinely be called a glucose sensor has been commercially available, in this case for measurement of capillary blood glucose levels (the 'Exactech pen', Medisense Ltd, Abingdon, Oxon, UK) – see Fig. 2. Implantable glucose sensors are reaching the stage of first clinical trials (Pickup *et al.*, 1989a), but it is generally agreed that they are many years from seeing application in routine patient care. Fig. 4 shows a prototype glucose sensor with a needle configuration, intended for implantation in the subcutaneous tissue of diabetic patients.

(e) An ex vivo sensor incorporated in a blood flow-through cell.

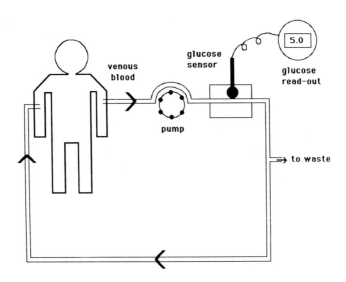

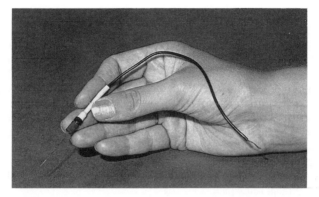

Figure 4. Prototype implantable glucose sensor. Glucose oxidase is immobilised in a polymer mixture on a platinum wire. Glucose concentration is proportional to the current recorded by the sensor.

Problems in the Development of Glucose Sensors

The apparently slow progress in this field makes an interesting case study in the development of medical technology, since it touches on the scientific, psychological and perhaps political hindrances that might exist in the translation of advanced technology to everyday medicine. Table 2 lists some obvious pre-requisites for the development and successful application of medical technology.

The need for a glucose sensor is well recognised by most doctors. The European Community Concerted Action on Chemical Sensors for In Vivo Monitoring, for example, sent a questionnaire during 1989 and 1990 to clinicians in 12 European countries, representing 18 specialities, and asked for details of clinical problems where continuous sensing would be appropriate. Diabetes mellitus was the most cited clinical problem, being mentioned about three times more often than the next most cited problem, the measurement of oxygenation in intensive care. Patients are probably equally clear about the need for glucose sensors, but their opinions do not seem formally to have been documented in this way.

Curiously, technologists are not always so certain about why a glucose sensor is being developed. Although a logical strategy for the introduction of a sensor should involve a sequence of questions (Table 3), beginning with 'What is the Clinical Problem?', this has been only rarely followed and may account in part for the slow progress. Often the reverse happens and work starts with a technology, or worse, just a scientific principle, for sensing. Hypoglycaemia, for example, is a completely different problem from the management of diabetes during surgery or the detection and prevention of ketoacidosis and these may demand different analyte measurements (glucose versus ketones), sensing sites (subcutaneous tissue versus blood), strategies (eg portable versus bedside apparatus), operating characteristics such as sampling frequency, linearity, response time etc, and thus different technologies. Here is an example of the difficulties of performing multidisciplinary science and the barriers to effective communication. Engineers and doctors are usually separated by their type of education, jargon and place of work, if nothing else.

There is often said to be an 'orgy' of available technology in the field of glucose sensing. Many hundreds of papers have been published describing methods for constructing glucose sensors (Turner and Pickup, 1985). The main reason why this profusion is at odds with the failure to produce clinical or commercial products is the fact that relatively little attention has been placed on making these many ingenious ideas work in practical situations. Implantable glucose sensors have faced at least four major difficulties which render the simple *in vitro* analysis of glucose solutions with such sensors of very little clinical relevance.

These problems are: the variation of the output of many sensors with alterations in oxygen levels at the sensing site, the need for *in vivo* calibration since sensors often give lower values when implanted than would be anticipated from prior *in vitro* calibration (Claremont *et al.,* 1986), the unpredictable drift of sensors *in vitro* and *in vivo*, and the perhaps related problem of the tissue-device interaction – biocompatibility.

Table 2

Some Requirements for the Development and Application of Medical Technology

A perceived need for the technology (identification of a clinical problem)
A logical development strategy
Appropriate available technology
Appropriate funding
Appropriate personnel

Table 3

A Logical Development Strategy for Biosensors

1. What is the clinical problem?
2. What analyte should be measured?
3. At what site in the body should the sensor measure (eg subcutaneous, intravenous etc)?
4. What should be the device strategy (eg warning alarm, feed-back control of drug etc)?
5. What should be the operating characteristics (eg linearity, sensitivity, reproducibility etc)?
6. In the light of the above, choose the appropriate technology.
7. Test in vitro and/or in vivo, modify as necessary and transfer to patient care.

Table 4

Negative Attitudes to High Technology

'Craft' (eg. engineering, technology, surgery, etc) is unscientific and just an
  application of science
Technology encourages unrealistic expectations, eg. diagnosis leads to
  effective treatment or therapy leads to cure
Technology is used routinely rather than selectively
Technology restricts lifestyle or movements
Technology distances the patient from the doctor
Technology is costly and/or a misuse of resources
Technology encourages academic rather than patient care aspects of medicine

Some progress has been made with several of these problems in recent
years. Oxygen sensitivity of sensors has been decreased by special covering
membranes (Gough *et al.*, 1985) and by the new technique of mediated
electron transfer, where oxygen is no longer the final electron acceptor in the
glucose oxidase-catalysed reaction, but electrons are directly transferred from
the enzyme to an underlying electrode (Cass *et al.*, 1984). Drift may also be
improved by tighter (covalent) attachment of glucose oxidase to electrodes
(Pickup *et al.*, 1989b). But the issues of biocompatibility and sensor
responses under various conditions in the tissues of normal subjects, let alone
diabetic patients, have hardly been touched.

Finally, assembling the skilled personnel and the necessary funding even
to begin to tackle the task (Table 2) has often also proved difficult. Perhaps
this is a reflection of our sometimes negative attitudes to High Technology
(Table 4). Of course, not all of these attitudes apply to glucose sensors, and
perhaps only a few people hold such views, but they are, nonetheless, well
known and long established. Some of these attitudes may be well-founded on
occasions. An artificial pancreas will not be a cure for diabetes, glucose
sensors should not be used indiscriminately in all diabetic patients – many
will resent being attached to a machine or may not have the type of diabetes
which would benefit from such a device. Development of sensors is certainly
costly and we need, therefore, as always, to ask searching questions about the
priorities for funding in diabetes research.

Summary and Conclusions

The diabetic patient can rightly claim that progress has been slow in the
development of glucose sensors and their application in devices such as an
artificial endocrine pancreas. Development has been partly frustrated by
technical factors such as instability of electrodes, variation of output with

changing oxygen tension and the interaction of implanted sensors with the
tissues. Some of these problems are now being actively addressed and *in vivo*
sensors are being tested for short periods of time in diabetic patients with
encouraging results. However, one might also argue that the hindrances to
progress reflect, to some degree, organisational and attitudinal difficulties in
medical technology. These include the need for multidisciplinary research,
the problem of achieving good communications between scientists of
different backgrounds and the logistics of providing expensive facilities in
many diverse fields of research. Negative attitudes towards medical
technology of this or other kinds, such as the view that it is costly, high-risk,
long-term and a possible misuse of resources, demands that its place in the
priorities of diabetes research is clearly set, and perhaps should be done so by
the patient as much as by the scientist or doctor.

References

Caras, S.D., Petelenz D.L. and Janata J. (1985). pH-based enzyme potentiometric
    sensors. Glucose-sensitive field effect transistor. *Analytic Chemistry* **57**,
    1920–1923.
Cass, A.E.G., Davies, G., Francis, C.D., Hill, H.A.D., Aston, W.J., Higgins, I.J. *et al.*
    (1984). Ferrocene-mediated enzyme electrode for amperometric determination of
    glucose. *Analytical Chemistry* **56**, 667–671.
Claremont, D.J., Sambrook, I.E., Penton, C and Pickup, J.C. (1986). Subcutaneous
    implantation of a ferrocene-mediated glucose sensor in pigs. *Diabetologia* **29**,
    817–821.
Clark, L.C. and Duggan, C.A., (1982). Implanted electroenzymatic glucose sensor.
    Diabetes Care **5**, 174–180.
Clark, L.C. and Lyons, C., (1962). Electrode systems for continuous monitoring in
    cardiovascular surgery. *Annals of the New York Academy of Science* **102**, 29–45.
Gough, D.A., Lucisana, J.Y. and Tse, P.H.S., (1985). Two-dimensional enzyme
    electrode sensor for glucose. *Analytical Chemistry* **57**, 2351–2357.
Heller, S.R., Macdonald, I.A., Herbert, M. and Tattersall, R.B., (1987). Influence of
    the sympathetic nervous system on hypoglycaemic warning symptoms. *Lancet* **ii**,
    359–363.
Lerner, H., Giner, J., Soeldner, J.S. and Cotton, L.K., (1984). An implantable
    electrochemical glucose sensor. *Annals of the New York Academy of Science* **428**,
    263–278.
Matthews, D.R., Holman, R.R., Bown, E., Steemson, J., Watson, A., Hughes, S. and
    Scott, D., (1987). Pen-sized digital 30-second blood glucose meter. *Lancet* **i**,
    778–779.
Pickup, J.C., (1985). Biosensors: a clinical perspective. *Lancet* **ii**, 817–820.
Pickup, J.C., Shaw, G.W. and Claremont, D.J., (1989a). In vivo molecular sensing in
    diabetes mellitus: an implantable glucose sensor with direct electron transfer.
    Diabetologia **32**, 213–217.
Pickup, J.C., Shaw, G.W. and Claremont, D.J., (1989b). *Potentially-implantable,
    amperometric* glucose sensors with mediated electron transfer: improving the
    operating stability. *Biosensors* **4**, 109–119.

Turner, A.P.F., Karube, I and Wilson, G.S., (Eds) (1987). *Biosensors: Fundamentals and Applications*. Oxford: Oxford University Press.

Turner, A.P.F. and Pickup J.C. (1985). Diabetes mellitus: biosensors for research and management. *Biosensors* **1**, 85–115.

Updike, S.J., and Hicks, J.P., (1967). The enzyme electrode. *Nature* **214**, 986–988.

Optimizing Blood Glucose Monitoring

Chris Gillespie

Department of Clinical Psychology, Pastures Hospital, Derby, UK

At the beginning of the 1980s self-monitoring of blood glucose (SMBG) in the management of diabetes was the subject of widespread and persistent optimism. Six research groups reported their experience with the blood glucose meters (Sonsken *et al.*, 1978; Walford *et al.*, 1978; Danowski and Sunder, 1978; Peterson *et al.*, 1978; Ikeda *et al.*, 1978; Skyler *et al.*, 1978). In a review of these reports, Tattersall (1980) concluded that: patients had little difficulty in pricking their fingers to obtain samples of capillary blood, the results were sufficiently accurate for clinical practice and that this method of direct self-monitoring led to increased motivation and better control in the majority of patients who made use of it.

Then Carney *et al.* (1981) followed by Shiffrin and Belmonte (1982) reported improved glycaemic control through SMBG. The technique was hailed as a crucial external feedback loop in the management of diabetes and was later endorsed by the American Diabetes Association (1987) which listed its advantages as:

1. SMBG provides individualised BG profiles to assist physician planning and decision making;
2. The technique facilitates appropriate day-to-day treatment choices by patients and their families;
3. It improves the recognition and prompt response to emergency situations (eg hypos);
4. It improves patient education by providing real-life demonstrations of principles learned in the classroom.

By the middle of the last decade, however, clinical experience with SMBG led Tattersall (1985) to conclude that long term SMBG would be monotonous and that patients were unlikely to follow the procedures diligently.

A similar reversal was apparent in the studies by Belmonte *et al.* (1988) and Mann *et al.* (1984) who found that the therapeutic promise of SMBG had not been widely delivered. It gradually emerged that the chain of events leading from the initiation of a blood glucose test to the effective use of the data implicated many behavioural and psychological variables. This had led to three lines of enquiry concerned with optimizing the impact of SMBG on metabolic control. Researchers have targeted either blood glucose data

38

collection or the subsequent use made of the data by patients. More recently, clinical studies have been reported suggesting that patients can learn to detect blood glucose levels. This learning process and the potential feedback mechanisms involved have generated a new field of enquiry now known as blood glucose discrimination.

Blood Glucose Data Collection

Prescribed SMBG routines probably consist of several independent behavioural dimensions, including the precision of the testing technique, reliability of SMBG diaries, the frequency of SMBG tests, or the scheduling of the tests.

Testing Technique or Precision

Clarke *et al.* (1987) provided the best evidence amongst dozens of studies which were designed to compare the accuracy of SMBG using correlations with laboratory results. They concluded that SMBG was generally quite precise in estimating BG levels and the data would result in correct treatment actions in 95 to 99% of instances. Clarson *et al.* (1985) found high correlations (r=0.89) between the SMBG of 90 children or their parents, but only 68% of the childrens results were within 20% of the laboratory results. There was no correlation between accuracy and metabolic control. Wing *et al.* (1985a) in a study of 280 children, SMBG results differed from the laboratory by a mean of 22.9%. Again, there was no correlation between accuracy and metabolic control.

The Patient Diary

Several recent studies have assessed the reliability of patient diaries by using results retrieved from meters with a memory function. Mazze *et al.* (1984) reported a significantly lower blood glucose mean in the patient's diaries that the mean stored in memory. The evidence suggested that patients added results (30.1%), or omitted results (8.3%) when comparing the diary record with memory. When both diary and memory recorded a test, there was disagreement in 25.7% of the cases. These findings were replicated by Lange and Mazze (1986) in a study of women with gestational diabetes. Phillips *et al.* (1987) studied 14 adults with diabetes unaware that their blood glucose meters had a memory function. When diary and meter results were compared, 64.3% of the patients were marginally or totally unreliable in diary recording.

Two studies have been reported showing the effects of making patients aware that their meters had a memory function. Mazze *et al.* (1985) demonstrated a rapid decrease of all kinds of errors but there was no significant change in the mean blood glucose concentration. Wilson and Endres (1986) studied 18 children with diabetes for six weeks unaware of the memory function and a further six weeks when they were informed that their results were being stored in memory. Errors were comparable to earlier studies though their reduction was less striking than that found by Mazze *et al.* (1985). In contrast Gonder-Frederick *et al.* (1986) found fewer diary errors in a study of 30 adults with insulin-treated diabetes though only 23% of patients presented diaries with no errors. In every case the memory function exerted little or no effect on metabolic control. Future studies using meters with memories need to be designed to explore the causes of recording bias provided the reliability of the memory function itself is also reported. In this way, the memory function would represent an effective behavioural assessment tool in diabetes care.

Blood Test Frequency

Testing frequency has been studied in both correlational (Hirsch *et al.*, 1983; Wing *et al.*, 1985b; Shiffrin and Belmonte 1982; Shafer *et al.* 1983; Glasgow *et al.*, 1987) and intervention studies (Smith *et al.*, 1985; Carney *et al.*, 1983; Wysocki *et al.*, 1988). The findings have generally been inconclusive and contradictory. Merely increasing SMBG data collection rates did not lead to changes in patient behaviour which could lead to improved metabolic control.

Scheduling of Tests

The distribution of tests across time according to a prescribed routine has been studied by Glasgow *et al.* (1987) who reported a compliance rate of 72%. This was not correlated with metabolic control.

Blood Glucose Data Utilisation

Knowledge of diabetes management, social and psychological factors, treatment actions based on SMBG data and the care process itself have been studied as potential influences on patient behaviour.

Knowledge of Diabetes Management

This literature has produced many inconsistent and contradictory findings, particularly where a single factor is predicted to enhance metabolic control. The exceptions to this rule are noteworthy. Wise *et al.* (1986) reported improved metabolic control, together with significant improvements in knowledge of diabetes. Bubb *et al.* (1987) found that training in self-management skills prevented deterioration of metabolic control when compared with conventional hospital procedures in 36 newly diagnosed children.

Social and Psychological Factors

Studies by Glasgow and Toobert (1988) and Delamatar *et al.* (1988) both found that the social context in which SMBG takes place may be an important factor in deciding outcome. In the first study family support predicted test frequency and, in the second, strong communication by health professionals for 'normal SMBG results' increased diary errors. Cox *et al.* (1985) found that patients were often guided in their treatment actions by beliefs about the relationship of symptoms to blood glucose levels. A large literature now exists on the predictive value of a range of patient beliefs on patient behaviour. Specific measures of diabetes-related health beliefs and perceptions of control have now been developed (Bradley *et al.*, 1984), and in a recent cross sectional study (Sjoberg *et al.*, 1988) significant correlations with metabolic control were reported. Future research is required using longitudinal designs and multivariate analysis since health care behaviour is probably the result of complex interactions between many psychological variables.

Treatment Actions based on SMBG Data

This important aspect of SMBG data utilisation has been largely neglected considering its crucial role in diabetes management. Four studies (Delamatar *et al.*, 1987; Hirsch *et al.*, 1983; Daneman *et al.*, 1982; Ingersoll *et al.*, 1986) all reported very low frequencies of clinical application of SMBG data. This applied particularly to insulin dose adjustment. However, Peyrot and Rubin (1988) found that patients who adjusted their own insulin or diet in response to SMBG were in better metabolic control. Greater attention needs to be paid to this variable in future research.

The clinical implications of these findings are that until we are able to mobilize the patient who can then feel confident and knowledgeable about appropriately responding to blood glucose test results, no changes can be expected in metabolic control.

The Care Process

Although many studies have been reported on the general nature of the physician-patient relationship, in only two studies has an aspect of the care process been associated with metabolic outcome. Using a cross-sectional design, Weinberger *et al.* (1984) compared groups of physicians for the success of two groups of physicians in caring for their patients, and found that their belief in the importance of strict metabolic control was reflected in the control obtained by their patients. More recently, Marteau and Kinmonth (1988) compared a group of general practitioners and hospital doctors and found that the former tolerated a wider range of blood glucose levels and were less convinced about the relationship between strict control and complications. These two studies demonstrate that the quality of control may be related to the attitudes of professional staff. Further studies are required comparing the effects of SMBG on metabolic control when staff attitudes are added to the equation.

It can be seen that data collection studies on their own provide little or no information on the quality of control. The studies of data utilisation, essential for changing metabolic control status, suggest that behavioural and psychological factors are implicated. The technology for measuring and storing blood glucose data, however reliable, cannot also provide the human behaviour required subsequently to respond to the information. Indeed, the evidence suggested that SMBG frequency alone does not influence long term blood glucose control. The medical ideal is so often in conflict with the individual's lifestyle that a low frequency of SMBG is the result (Hirsch *et al.*, 1983). One solution to this problem is suggested by the third line of enquiry involving blood glucose discrimination training which may be more compatible with the patients lifestyle.

Blood Glucose Discrimination Training

Through the use of systematic feedback individuals have been taught to detect various psysiological functions like peripheral temperature (Gillespie and Peck, 1980), heart rate (Brener and Jones, 1974), blood pressure (Luborsky *et al.*, 1976) and blood alcohol levels (Vogel-Sprott, 1975). As a result of these earlier successes, these principles can be applied to the use of systematic blood glucose feedback in order to teach blood glucose discrimination.

Two concepts in psychology guided this kind of research. Firstly, feedback itself is one of the most profound and unifying concepts in the behavioural sciences. When used systematically, individuals have been taught to detect various physiological functions like peripheral temperature, heart rate, blood pressure and blood alcohol levels. As a result of these earlier successes, these principles can be applied to SMBG in order to teach BG discrimination. This would allow patients to perceive blood glucose levels subjectively and continuously. When this skill is accompanied by intermittent SMBG to validate subjective estimates, the whole selfmonitoring procedure would be more compatible with the patient's lifestyle.

Secondly, the concept of self-monitoring in psychology has provided many demonstrations of its useful self-regulatory functions (Thoreson and Mahoney, 1974). The advances in technology which have made SMBG a reality for many patients, also provide the basic procedures that would be required for blood glucose discrimination training. Accurate self monitoring of the appropriate physiological variable permits the patient to acquire the new skill of blood glucose discrimination. In particular, if patients could learn to detect blood glucose levels outside the normoglycaemic range, then SMBG could be used more effectively without adding to the burdens of self-management.

Three important general questions need to be asked before examining the available literature. Firstly, can individuals with diabetes without special training detect blood glucose levels with any accuracy? Secondly, can the ability to detect BG levels be significantly improved by a feedback training strategy? Thirdly, will this improved skill lead to significant improvement in the ability to control blood sugars within the normal range? In trying to find answers to questions like these, a very fertile field of research has been opened up in BG discrimination training strategies.

The first question had emerged from the belief shared by many patients that they could estimate their own blood glucose levels by noting their physical symptoms. This possibility was investigated by Pennebaker *et al.* (1981) who found some correlations between estimated blood glucose and symptoms but concluded that glucose estimation without training or constant recourse to SMBG would lead to serious treatment errors. A serious note of caution has been issued about the inadvisability of instructing individual patients to attend to and respond to standard symptoms (Cox *et al.*, 1985).

The second question was widely addressed and the consensus was that blood glucose estimation errors could be reduced with feedback procedures of various kinds. A large range of individual differences in the ability to acquire the new skill were reported. Feedback procedures themselves differed. In some interventions the patients received no instructions of how feedback could be best used and in others they received detailed instructions. When instructed, patients were required to selectively attend to internal or external cues. It remains unknown which cues (if any) or combination of cues were used by patients in the uninstructed feedback procedures. In addition, instructions varied in the way cues were to be used. Instructions to attend to internal mood state cues, at the time of blood glucose estimation, led Bradley and Jeffries (1980) and Moses and Bradley (1985) to the conclusion that feedback could operate effectively via internal cues.

Gillespie (1989) compared two feedback strategies. In a study involving 20 adult, insulin-treated outpatients, Gillespie (1989) compared two feedback strategies. The first group (mean age 39.7 years; mean duration of diabetes 16.9 years) was instructed to use mood state cues in order to estimate blood glucose levels. The second group (mean age 46.0 years; mean duration of diabetes 18.7 years) was given no instructions on how to use SMBG feedback. A wide range of individual differences masked any between group effects on estimation accuracy. Approximately half the individuals in each group improved their discrimination. In clinical practice an assessment could be made as to which set of cues have discriminative value for each individual. These can then be used for daily self-management. Intermittent recourse to a blood glucose meter could then serve to validate these estimates. An optimum strategy for any one individual may be a combination of particular internal and external cues. Table I provides a summary of clinical studies aimed at improving estimation accuracy in various settings and the feedback strategies used or implied.

Table 1 *Clinical studies demonstrating blood glucose estimation error,*
feedback strategies implied and setting employed.

Study	Feedback Mechanisms	Setting
Bradley & Jeffries, 1980	FIC; mood state	Home
Gross *et al.*, 1983	F (external assumed)	Hospital
Cameron *et al.*, 1980	FIC; symptoms	Hospital
Gross *et al.*, 1984	F (external assumed)	Hospital
Moses & Bradley, 1985	FIC; effects of delay	Home
Gross *et al.*, 1985	F (external assumed)	Hospital
Cox *et al.*, 1985	FIC vs FEC (+FIC?)	Both
Roales-Nieto, 1988	FEC vs F (random)	Hosital
Gillespie, 1989	FIC Effect of instructions	Home

FIC, feedback internal cue
FEC, feedback external cue
F, feedback

The third question which related to the effect of improved estimation accuracy on blood glucose control has barely been addressed although the rationale for improved estimation was based on the potential for improved blood glucose control. There was no evidence that estimation error reduction was associated with improvement in HbA_1 (a measure of long term blood glucose control) in patients with poor control.

Summary and Conclusion

It becomes clear that evidence from all three lines of enquiry need to be carefully considered when calculating the usefulness of further developments in the technology of blood glucose data collection devices. Usefulness usually implies an improved metabolic outcome, but there are other short-term outcomes in diabetes care associated with the quality of life. Glucose sensors would clearly benefit those patients who were unable to learn blood glucose discrimination skills. This would then permit better patient selection when evaluating the usefulness of glucose sensors.

In the meantime, the appropriate use of blood glucose data which may include insulin dose adjustment, provides the most potent mechanism for enhancing metabolic control. This will ultimately decide the usefulness of BG data collection technology. Detailed reliable assessments of knowledge of diabetes, beliefs about the value of diabetes management and perceptions of control are most likely to reveal the nature and size of the individual differences to be expected in making effective use of gathered blood glucose data. There is also growing evidence that the attitudes and beliefs of staff may play a role in deciding patient outcomes. Only data of this kind can inform us of what sense is being made by patients of SMBG data. Advances in the technology of BG data collection will be limited in their usefulness until the patient is able to actively participate in their use, which would need to be seen as a logical extension of their own resources for the management of their diabetes.

References

American Diabetes Association (1987) Consensus statement on self-monitoring of blood glucose. *Diabetes Care* 10: 95– 99.

Belmonte, M., Schiffrin, A., Dufresne, J., Suissa, S., Goldman, H., and Polychronakos, C. (1988) Impact of SMBG on control of diabetes as measured by HbA$_1$: A 3 year survey of a juvenile IDDM clinic. *Diabetes Care* 11, 484–488.

Bradley, C., Brewin, C.R., Gamsu, D.S., Moses, J.L., (1984) Development of scales to measure perceived control of diabetes mellitus and diabetes-related health beliefs. *Diabetic Medicine* 1, 133–146.

Bradley, C., and Jeffries, S.C. (1980) Autofeedback in the management of diabetes. *Biological Psychology* 11 (3/4), 277.

Brener, J., and Jones, J.M. (1974) Interoceptive discrimination in intact humans: detection of cardiac activity. *Physiology and Behaviour* 13, 763.

Bubb, J., Delamater, A.M., Smith, J., and White, N. (1987) Effects of self management training (SMT) on metabolic control of children with newly diagnosed diabetes: A one year follow up. *Diabetes* 36 (Suppl. 1), 86A.

Cameron, O.G. and Curtis, G.C. (1980) Discrimination of intravenously administered glucose by non-diabetic humans. *Psychomatic Medicine* 42 (1), 73.

Carney, R.M., Schechter, K., Homa, M., Levandoski, L., White N., and Santiago, J. (1981) The effects of blood glucose testing versus urine glucose testing on the metabolic control of insulin-dependent diabetic children. *Diabetes Care* 4, 378–380.

Carney, R.M., Schechter, K., and Davis, T., (1983) Improving adherence to blood glucose testing in insulin-dependent diabetic children. *Behaviour Therapy* 14, 247–254.

Clarke, W.L., Cox, D.J., Gonder-Frederick, L.M., Carter, W., and Pohl, S. (1987) Evaluating the clinical accuracy of systems for self-monitoring of blood glucose. *Diabetes Care* 10, 622–628.

Clarson, C., Daneman, D., Frank, M., Link, J., Perlman, K., and Ehrlich, R.M. (1985). self-monitoring of blood glucose: How accurate are children with diabetes at reading Chemstrip BG? *Diabetes Care* 8, 354–358.

Cox, D.J., Clarke, W.L., and Gonder-Frederick, L.M. (1985). Accuracy of perceiving blood glucose in IDDM. *Diabetes Care* 8, 529–536.

Cox, D.J., Gonder-Frederick, L.A., Pohl, S., *et al.* (1983) Reliability of symptom-blood glucose relationships among insulin-dependent adult diabetics. *Psychosomatic Medicine* 45, 357–360.

Cox, D.J., Gonder-Frederick, L.A., Pohl, S. *et al.* (1985) Symptoms and blood glucose levels in diabetics. *Journal of the American Medical Association* 253, 1558.

Daneman, D., Epstein, L.H., Siminerio, L., Beck, S., Farkas, G., Figueroa, J., Becker, D.J., and Drash, A.L. (1982) Effects of enhanced conventional therapy on metabolic control in children with insulin-dependent diabetes mellitus. *Diabetes Care* **5**, 472–478.

Danowski, T.S., Sunder, J.H. (1978) Jet injection of insulin during self-monitoring of of blood glucose. *Diabetes Care* **1**, 27–33.

Delamatar, A.M., Davis, S.G., Bubb, J., and Smith, J. (1987) Utilization of self blood glucose monitoring (SMBG) data by adolescents with diabetes. (Abstract) *Diabetes* **36** (Suppl. 1), 17A.

Gillespie, C.R. and Peck, D.F. (1980) The effects of biofeedback and guided imagery on finger temperature. *Biological Psychology* **11**, 235–247.

Gillespie, C.R. (1989) Psychological Variables in the Self Regulation of Diabetes Mellitus. PhD Thesis. University of Sheffield, England.

Glasgow, R.E., McCaul, K.D., and Schafer, L. (1987) Self care behaviours and glycemic control in Type I diabetes. *Journal of Chronic Diseases* **40**, 399–412.

Glasgow, R.E., and Toobert, D.J. (1988) Social environment and regime adherence among Type II diabetic patients. *Diabetes Care* **11**, 377–386.

Gonder-Frederick, L., Julian, D.M., Cox, D.J., Clarke, W.L., and Carter, W. (1988) Self-measurement of blood glucose: Accuracy of self reported data and adherence to recommended regimen. *Diabetes Care* **11**, 579–585.

Gross, A.M., Wojnilower, D.A., Levin, R.B., *et al.* (1983) Discrimination of blood glucose levels in insulin dependent diabetics. *Behaviour Modification* **7**, 369–382.

Gross, A.M., Levin, R.B., Mulvihill, M. *et al.* (1984) Blood glucose discrimination training with insulin dependent diabetics: A clinical note. *Biofeedback and Self Regulation* **9**, 49–54.

Gross, A.M., MacGalnick, L.J., and Delcher, H.J. (1985) Blood glucose discrimination training and metabolic control in insulin dependent diabetics. *Behavioural Research and Therapy* **23**, 507–511.

Hirsch, I., Matthews, M., Rawlings, S. *et al.* (1983) Home capillary blood glucose monitoring (HBGM) for diabetic youth: A one year follow up of 98 patients. (Abstract) *Diabetes* **32** (Suppl. 1) 16A.

Ikeda, Y., Tajima, N., Nimani, N., Ide, Y. *et al.* (1978) Pilot study of self measurement of blood glucose using the Dextrostix-Eyetone System for juvenile onset diabetes. *Diabetologia* **15**, 91–93.

Ingersoll, G., Orr, D., Herrold, A., and Golden, M. (1986) Cognitive maturity and self management among adolescents with insulin-dependent diabetes mellitus. *Journal of Paediatrics* **108**, 620–623.

Langer, O., and Mazze, R.S. (1986) Diabetes in pregnancy: Evaluating self-monitoring Performance and glycemic control with memory-based reflectance meters. *American Journal of Obstetrics and Gynecology* **155**, 635–637.

Luborsky, L., Brady, J.P., McClintock, M. *et al.* (1976) Estimating one's own ststolic blood pressure. Effects of feedback training. *Psychosomatic Medicine* **38**, 426–438.

Mann, N.P., Noronha, J.L. and Johnston, D.I. (1984). A prospective study to evaluate the benefits of long term self monitoring of blood glucose in diabetic children. *Diabetes Care* **7**, 322–326.

Marteau, T.M., and Kinmonth, A.L. (1988) Doctors' beliefs about diabetes: A comparison of hospital and community doctors. *British Journal of Clinical Psychology* **27**, 381–383.

Mazze, R.S., Shamoon, H., Pasmantier, R., Lucido, D., Murphy, J., Hartmann, K., Kuykendall, V., and Lopatin, W. (1984) Reliability of blood glucose monitoring by patients with diabetes mellitus. *American Journal of Medicine* **77**, 211–217.

Mazze, R.S., Pasmantier, R., Murphy, J., and Shamoon, H. (1985) Self monitoring of capillary blood glucose: Changing the performance of individuals with diabetes. *Diabetes Care* **8**, 207–213.

Moses, J.L., and Bradley, C. (1985) Accuracy of subjective blood glucose estimation by patients with insulin dependent diabetes. *Biofeedback and Self-Regulation* **10**, 4, 301–314.

Pennebaker, J.W., Cox, D.J., Gonder-Frederick, L.A. (1981) Physical symptoms related to blood glucose in insulin dependent diabetics. *Psychosomatic Medicine* **43**, 488 500.

Peterson, C.M., Jones, R.L., Dupuis, A., *et al.* (1978) Feasibility of tight control of juvenile diabetes through patient monitored glucose determinations. *Diabetes* **27** (suppl. 2), 437.

Peyrot, M., and Rubin, R.R. (1988) Insulin self regulation predicts better glycemic control. (Abstract) *Diabetes* **37** (Suppl. 1), 53A.

Phillips, R., Sanchez, J., Pedromingo, A., and Fernandez-Cruz, A. (1987) An evaluation of the credibility of blood glucose results reported by diabetic patients through the use of a reflectance meter with memory. (Abstract) *Diabetes* **36**, (suppl. 1), 63A.

Roales-Neito, J.G. (1988) Blood glucose discrimination in insulin dependent diabetics: Training in feedback and external cues. *Behaviour Modification* **12**, No. 1, 116–132.

Shafer, L.C., Glasgow, R.E., McCaul, K.D. and Dreher, M. (1983) Adherence to IDDM regimens: Relationship to psychological variables and metabolic control. *Diabetes Care* **6** 493–498.

Shiffrin, A., and Belmonte, M. (1982) Multiple daily self glucose monitoring: Its essential role in long term glucose control in insulin-dependent diabetic patients treated with pump and multiple subcutaneous injections. *Diabetes Care* **9**, 479–484.

Sjoberg, S., Carlson, A., Rosenqvist, U., and Ostman, J. (1988) Health attitudes self-monitoring of blood glucose, metabolic control and residual insulin secretion in type I diabetic patients. *Diabetic Medicine* **5**, 449–453.

Skyler, J.S., Lasky, I.A., Kkyler, D.L., *et al.* (1978) Home blood glucose monitoring as an aid in diabetes management. *Diabetes Care* **1**, 150–157.

Smith, M.A., Greene, S., Kuykendall, V., and Baum, J. (1985) Memory blood glucose reflectance meter and computer: A preliminary report of its use in recording and analyzing blood glucose data measured at home by diabetic children. *Diabetic Medicine* **2**, 265–268.

Sonsken, P.H., Judd, S L. and Lowry, C. (1978) Home monitoring of blood glucose: Method for improving diabetic control. *Lancet* **1**, 729–732.

Tattersall, R.B. (1980) Workshop on Home Monitoring of Blood-Glucose. Internal Publication. Nottingham University, Nottingham, England.

Tattersall, R.B. (1985) Self monitoring of blood glucose. 1978–1984. *Diabetes Annual* **1**. Eds K.G.M.M. Alberti and L.P. Krall. Amsterdam Elsevier.

Thoreson, C.E., and Mahoney, M.J. (1974) *Behavioural Self-Control.* New York: Holt, Rinehart and Winston.

Vogel-Sprott, M. (1975) Self-evaluations of performance and the ability to discriminate blood alcohol concentrations. *Journal of Studies on Alcohol* **36**, 1–10.

Walford, S., Gale, E.A.M., Allison, S.P. and Tattersall R.B. (1978) Self-monitoring of blood glucose. *Lancet* **1**, 732–735.

Weinberger, M., Cohen, S.J., and Mazzuca, S.A. (1984) The role of physician's knowledge and attitudes in effective diabetes management. *Social Science and Medicine* **19**, 965–968.

Wilson, D.P., and Endres, R.K. (1986) Compliance with blood glucose monitoring in children with Type I diabetes mellitus. *Journal of Pediatrics* **108**, 1022–1024.

Wing, R., Lamparski, D., Zaslow, S., Betschart, J., Siminerio, L., and Becker, D. (1985a) Frequency and accuracy of self monitoring of blood glucose in children: Relationship to glycemic control. *Diabetes Care* **7**: 476–478.

Wing, R., Koeske, R., New, A., Lamparski, D., and Becker, D. (1985b) Compliance to self monitoring of blood glucose: A marked item technique compared with self report. *Diabetes Care* **8**, 456–460.

Wise, P.H., Dowlatshi, D., Farrant, S., Fromson, S., and Meadows, K. (1986) Effect of computer-based learning on diabetes knowledge and control. *Diabetes Care* **9**, 504–508.

Wysocki, T., Green, L., and Huxtable, K., (1988) Behavioural application of reflectance meters with memory in juvenile diabetes. (Abstract) *Diabetes* **37** (Suppl. 1), 18A.

The Use of a Computerised System in a Diabetic Pregnancy Clinic

Huw Alban Davies

Consultant Diabetologist, West Hill Hospital, Dartford, Kent. DA1 2HF, UK.

Introduction

The outcome of diabetic pregnancy depends on the quality of blood glucose control at the time of conception and during gestation (Karlsson and Kjellmer 1972, Miller *et al.*, 1981, Watkins 1982). Other factors, including the age of onset of diabetes and the presence of complications of diabetes are less important (Jovanovic *et al.*, 1981). In the last 40 years, by means of progressive improvements in blood glucose control, it has been possible to reduce the rates of congenital abnormality and perinatal mortality from as high as 15% and 40% respectively to a figure no greater than that of non-diabetic pregnancies (Karlsson and Kjellmer 1972, Jovanovic *et al.*, 1981, Fuhrmann *et al.*, 1983).

To achieve what was regarded as the optimal standard of contemporary blood glucose control different management was required in different decades. Until about 1980 all pregnant diabetic women were admitted to hospital at about 28 weeks gestation so that meticulous control could be enforced with the assistance of laboratory blood glucose measurements. In the last decade the use of reagent strips for measuring blood glucose has become widely accepted (Fuhrmann *et al.*, 1983). With strips, self blood glucose monitoring has become feasible and it is now possible to achieve satisfactory results in pregnancy without routine admission to hospital during the final trimester (Jovanovic *et al.*, 1980). Pregnant women at home are able to measure their own blood glucose more often than was possible in hospital and the main difference between the two regimens is that the women themselves take on more reponsibility for their condition. During the course of a diabetic pregnancy the patient must carry out a large number of tests on herself and make many alterations in her own insulin regimen. Information technology has the potential to be used for the patient's benefit in this situation. In particular, it can help to analyse blood glucose data and to assess performance towards defined goals.

49

Measurements of blood glucose are carried out by means of hand-held reflectance meters. These meters can be fitted out with microcircuitary capable of timing and memorising up to 440 measurements of blood glucose (Glucometer-M, Ames Division, Miles Industries, Elkhart, Ind.,USA). The data are later uploaded on to a clinic-based microcomputer and can be presented in a number of graphic and numerical formats to assist with education and diabetes control. Data are manipulated to give the following parameters. Average blood glucose level is computed between specified dates;

1. for all readings,
2. within 6-hour periods and,
3. on each day of the week.

Another format displays all the individual blood glucose values plotted on a single 24-hour cycle. Target ranges for blood glucose can be set and the percentage of readings falling above, below and within this range given. The target range could be altered according to the clnical situation, so that patients with a tendency to hypoglycaemia could be set a higher range than those without. Individual readings are also displayed graphically by the time of day, in a diary format.

The optimal environment for clinical management of diabetic pregnancy is the joint medical-obstetric clinic because it allows an integrated approach to common problems and the patient needs to make fewer visits to hospital. The use of computerised systems fits readily into this context and I have been involved with a "computerised" diabetic pregnancy clinic for six years. This was initially at the Rosie Maternity Hospital, Cambridge and more lately at the Maternity Unit, Gravesend and North Kent Hospital. Insulin dependent diabetic women are supplied with Glucometer-Ms (G-Ms) at the time they book into the maternity service or when they decide to attempt a pregnancy (pre-conception care). Blood glucose readings are taken in the same way as with a standard meter but data are later transferred from the G-M's memory chip to a clinic-based IBM-PC microcomputer, by means of an RS 232 interface. A total of 33 diabetic women have now used the G-M system .

Experience

Experience of the first 24 women using the computerised system in Cambridge shows that it is possible to maintain virtual euglycaemia by the end of the pregnancy. The average age of the women was 28 (SD 4) yr, and they were enrolled into the clinic at 11 (5) weeks gestation. Delivery occurred at 38.8 (1.5) weeks. An average of 4.4 (1.2) readings were made per patient per day during their pregnancies. Average blood glucose values in the first, second and third trimesters were respectively 6.7 (1.1), 6.4 (1.2) and 5.9 (0.9) mmol/l. There was no correlation between frequency of blood glucose testing and mean blood glucose levels. Corresponding values for HbA_1 were 7.8 (1.5), 6.4 (0.9) and 6.2 (0.7) %. All women delivered healthy babies.

An attempt was made to involve patients in the data analysis by sitting them in front of the computer screen and asking for their comments about the displays. Most patients could readily identify trends towords hyper- and hypoglycaemia, and of poor timing between insulin injection and food; they were encouraged to suggest insulin dose alterations on the basis of this analysis. During the course of the pregnancy the average daily insulin dose increased from 45 (14) to 91(33) units per day, the greatest dose increments occuring between 20 and 36 weeks gestation. In certain cases women found that they responded to the incentive of target-chasing, when they tried to increase the percentage of readings within the target range. Thirteen of these pregnant women were asked their opinion about the G-M system. Of these, 82% considered it helpful and the chief reason given was that it increased confidence in management by making the most of the available information, while 18% felt that it added little to logbook inspection.

When the G-M system was used in the diabetic pregnancy clinic in Gravesend the same basic method was followed. Although it was not possible to have such close collaboration with obstetricians, a closer liason was formed between pregnant women and diabetes specialist nurses. The first 9 women managed at Gravesend were well matched with the Cambridge group so far as age, gestation at booking and duration of diabetes were concerned. Their average blood glucose values for the 1st, 2nd and 3rd trimesters were 8.8 (2), 7.2 (1) and 6.8 (1.1) mmol/l respectively; the 1st and 3rd trimester values were significantly higher than in the Cambridge group (t-test, $p<0.05$). The fall in average blood glucose values between 1st and 3rd trimesters for the Gravesend group was 23% and this was nearly twice the fall for the Cambridge group (12%).

Six of the pregnant women in the Cambridge clinic transmitted blood glucose data from their own homes using their G-M and a telephone modem. In this way the timed readings were sent to the clinic-based microcomputer telemetrically, by means of a telephone land line. After the readings had been input to the microcomputer the diabetologist explained the analysis to the patient and discussed her diabetes control by telephone. A total of 42 transmissions were made in this way and the patients were saved the inconvenience and expense of travelling to hospital on these occasions.

Discussion

The use of G-Ms is practical, convenient and well accepted by patients. Their use has been shown to lead to more accurate reporting of blood glucose by patients in their own logbooks. Mazze (1984) found that 26% of all readings entered in logbooks were inaccurate, with a tendency for poor readings to be omitted or 'improved'; when subjects were told that their standard glucose meters had been substituted by G-Ms the accuracy of reporting increased

(Mazze *et al.*, 1985). However they found that metabolic control, as judged by HbA₁ measurements, did not improve when computerised systems were used, despite more accurate reporting by patients. This observation may be related to the insensitivity of objective tests for assessing diabetic control; HbA_1 reflects mean blood glucose, and wide excursions above and below the mean cancel each other out. The tendency for patients to present an idealised view of their metabolic control appears to be greater in pregnancy than at other times. Logbooks of 66% of a group of non-pregnant patients were inaccurate, but when the exercise was repeated in a group of pregnant patients, 80% of them were shown to be inaccurate; in these studies the patients were unaware that their meters had a memory facility (Langer and Mazze 1986).

Computerised systems are particularly helpful in pregnancy because of the large number of readings involved. Women took on average 4.4 blood glucose readings per day; between booking at 11 weeks and delivery at 39 weeks no less than 848 readings were taken per patient and to analyse these data by studying the logbook would have been a major undertaking. Our patients derived confidence from the computerised analysis, feeling that the most was made of their considerable efforts.

Average blood glucose is a useful criterion for decision-making in a diabetic pregnancy clinic. Target values can be set for the woman who wants to optimise control before conceiving. Also, during pregnancy a blood glucose range can be set with the agreement that should the weekly average deviate beyond an agreed threshold, hospital admission is then required for close supervision. When used in this way blood glucose statistics are intrinsically preferable to HbA_1. HbA_1 is retrospective with a lag-time of approximately 5 weeks in pregnancy whereas management decisions in diabetic pregnancy are more pressing than this time frame allows. With M-G analysis performance can be reviewed on a weekly basis and decisions made accordingly, but it is not useful to repeat the HbA_1 at less than one month intervals. It is true that logbook entries can be used to calculate mean blood glucose but this is time consuming and not practical in the clinical situation.

In this study the G-M system was used to help in the management of diabetic pregnancy; no comparison has been made with a standard system in which control is monitored by inspecting the patient's own record, the blood glucose logbook. The system has been used in two different clinics situated in different parts of the country. Although the average blood glucose obtained by Cambridge women was significantly lower than by those in Gravesend, the Gravesend women achieved a relatively larger fall in their average blood glucose during pregnancy. The reason for the differences in diabetes control between patients living in the two areas can only be speculated upon. Cambridge has a relatively greater proportion of highly skilled workers who may be familiar with technological advances and this may have an effect on their ability to manage their own diabetes successfully. It did not seem to be the case that the Gravesend women were any less motivated than the Cambridge group; clinic attendances and commitment were extremely high in both places. Other factors are also likely to have an influence on the quality of diabetes control. The amount of time available for diabetes self-care was not investigated nor was the effect that other children at home may have had on their mothers.

The most important difference between the control of blood glucose in pregnancy and at other times is the the immediate relationship between the result achieved and the outcome. The pregnant woman is aware of the consequences of poor control for her own pregnancy and she is often anxious about her own performance. Questionnaire findings from women in this study suggested that the use of G-M led to increased confidence, but it would be valuable to carry out a formal comparison looking not only at the quality of metabolic control but also the psychological wellbeing, satisfaction with treatment and convenience for the pregnant woman in terms of the number of visits to clinic and time spent in hospital. Other health outcomes such as the duration of pregnancy, method of delivery and wellbeing of mother and child may be influenced by the means used to achieve diabetes control but there are a large number of other factors which also influence these outcomes.

This was a pilot study in the use of telephone modems for monitoring diabetes control. Telemetry of results from home to hospital has great potential to reduce the number of clinic visits without affecting the degree of super-vision. However, in the pilot stage a large number of visits to the patient's home were required to ensure that the equipment functioned and that women were able to master the technology. It is likely that blood glucose telemetry could be introduced as a routine service with very little supervision, with the experience gained from these womens' use of the system.

In conclusion, a computerised system has been used in a diabetes antenatal clinic to analyse the large number of blood glucose readings that each woman is required to make during pregnancy. Women did not appear to find the computer intrusive and it gave them confidence in the management of their diabetes. The telemetric relay of blood glucose data from the pregnant woman's own home promises considerable convenience in terms of time saved attending and travelling to clinic, although in this pilot study the successful relay of data involved quite considerable outlay of time by staff. When used in clinic the G-M system did not lead to any significant disruption of the clinic routine and there was no delay involved with uploading data to the computer and studying the analysis. Metabolic control in pregnancy is vital to outcome and if blood glucose is brought into the normal range diabetes can be eliminated as a risk factor for congenital abnormality and perinatal mortality. The G-M system allows an accurate audit of the state of metabolic control and any lapse in the high standard required can be detected without delay.

54   HUW ALBAN DAVIES

References

Fuhrmann K, Reicher H, Semmler K, Fischer F, Fischer M, Glockner E. (1983). Prevention of congenital malformations in infants of insulin-dependent mothers. *Diabetes Care* **6**, 219–223.

Jovanovic L, Peterson CM, Saxena BB, Dawood MY, Saudek CD. (1980). Feasibility of maintaining normal glucose profiles in insulin-dependent pregnant diabetic women. *American Journal of Medicine* **68**, 105–112.

Jovanovic L, Druzin M, Peterson CM. (1981). Effect of euglycaemia on the outcome of pregnancy in insulin dependent diabetic women as compared with normal subjects. *American Journal of Medicine* **71**, 921–927.

Karlsson K, Kjellmer I. (1972). The outcome of diabetic pregnancies in relation to the mother's blood sugar level. *American Journal of Obstetrics and Gynecology* **112**, 213–220.

Langer O, Mazze RS. (1986). Diabetes in pregnancy: evaluating self-monitoring performance and glycaemic control with memory-based reflectance meters. *American Journal of Obstetrics and Gynecology* **155**, 635–637.

Mazze RS, Shamoon H, Pasmantier R, Lucido D, Murphy J, Hartmann K, Kuykendal V, Lopatin W. (1984). Reliability of blood glucose monitoring by patients with diabetes mellitus. *American Journal of Medicine* **77**, 211–217.

Mazze RS, Pasmantier R, Murphy J, Shamoon H. (1985). Self-monitoring of capillary blood glucose: changing performance of individuals with diabetes. *Diabetes Care* **8**, 207–213

Miller E, Hare JW, Cloherty JP, Dunn PJ, Gleason RE, Soeldner S, Kitzmiller JL. (1981). Elevated maternal Hemoglobin A1c in early pregnancy and major congenital abnormalities in infants of diabetic mothers. *New England Journal of Medicine* **304**, 1331–1334.

Watkins PJ. (1982). Congenital malformations and blood glucose control in diabetic pregnancy. *British Medical Journal* **284**, 1357–1358.

2

INSULIN AND INSULIN DELIVERY

Recent developments in genetic engineering using recombinant DNA technology have opened the way for commercial production of 'human insulin'. Insulin supply is thus assured. However, human insulin may not be without its problems. In some patients, transfer from animal to human insulin is associated with apparent loss of the warning symptoms of hypoglycaemia. This association, which may be causal, indirectly related or coincidental, has provided further stimulus to research on insulin-induced hypoglycaemia reviewed in the following chapter by David Hepburn and Brian Frier.. Investigations have involved the development of physiological and hormonal indicators to identify the onset and magnitude of autonomic activation in individual patients and the use of neuropsychological tests to assess the effects of lowered blood glucose concentration on the brain. This area of research has brought together medical and psychological perspectives to the study of phenomena where individual differences between patients, symptoms and their experience of those symptoms, are profound.

The following two chapters are both concerned with methods of insulin delivery. The first, by Philip Home, describes the development of inplantable insulin infusion pumps. Externally worn continuous subcutaneous insulin infusion pumps have been considered by several contributors elsewhere in this book (Keen, Marteau, Bradley). Surgically implanted insulin pumps are the variety of pump considered here by Home. The technical, medical, psychological and economic problems faced in the process of developing such pumps are described; many of these problems appear insuperable. In order to justify the use of the risky, disfiguring and expensive technology currently available, the diabetes would need to be in such poor control that quality and quantity of life were seriously threatened. Yet patients in this position, with so-called brittle diabetes, are often believed to have psychological problems which cause or exacerbate their metabolic problems with their diabetes. The difficulties involved in tackling the problems of implantable insulin pumps are likely to be magnified when pumps are implanted in patients with such complex problems.

In theory it might be assumed that surgically implanted pumps would relieve the patient of responsibility for managing their diabetes, while the technology and technologists take control. The reality proves to be quite different, with the patient required to operate a remote control device with all the dangers of interference and error, electronic and human.

C

At the other extreme of insulin delivery devices are the pen-injectors designed to be as portable as a pen and almost as easy to use. Pen-injectors were designed to facilitate patients' control of their diabetes and life style. Pen-injectors are the subject of the chapter by Judith North who considers the impact of these devices on the lives of the mostly young people who use them. The real potential in pen-injectors has not been in their promise for improved diabetes control but in their providing an easier way of administering insulin that allows greater flexibility of life style without loss of blood glucose control. If, in clinical trials evaluating the use of pen-injectors, the only outcomes measured are metabolic outcomes and financial costs, the pen-injector is not shown to advantage compared with the conventional syringe. When, however, various components of quality of life are among the outcomes investigated, the pen-injector is found to have a much better chance of demonstrating its potential. Technologies such as pen-injectors are likely to benefit from more holistic evaluation of the kind considered in the chapters by Bradley and by Meadows in the last section of this book.

The Use of Technology in Assessing Manifestations of Acute Insulin-Induced Hypoglycaemia in Humans

David A. Hepburn and Brian M. Frier
Department of Diabetes, Royal Infirmary, Edinburgh, EH3 9YW, Scotland, UK.

Hypoglycaemia

In humans blood glucose is maintained within a narrow range by various homeostatic mechanisms; hypoglycaemia occurs when the blood glucose is reduced below this normal range. Although defined biochemically as an arterial blood glucose below 2.2 mmol/l, many clinical features of hypoglycaemia can be detected at blood glucose concentrations above this value. The investigation of many aspects of acute hypoglycaemia, in the laboratory and in the community, depends on the use of technology to assess the hormonal, physiological and symptomatic responses. Many of the techniques used are being developed to assist the investigation of abnormal hypoglycaemic episodes in patients with insulin-dependent diabetes mellitus. Hypoglycaemia is the commonest adverse reaction to the routine administration of insulin to diabetic patients and is potentially the most serious. It is associated with a significant morbidity and mortality (Frier, 1986). When glycaemic control in diabetic patients is optimized with intensification of insulin regimens the frequency of hypoglycaemia may be increased. In one large trial (described by Kramer and Colleagues in Section 4) the frequency of severe hypoglycaemia has been reported to be 2–3 times higher than with conventional therapy (The DCCT Research Group, 1987), although this has not been found in other studies.

Physiological Background

The onset of hypoglycaemia both in non-diabetic and diabetic individuals is associated with the development of two groups of symptoms: (1) NEUROGLYCOPENIC symptoms and (2) AUTONOMIC symptoms. Glucose cannot be stored or synthesized by the central nervous system; the dependence of the brain on the oxidative metabolism of glucose as its source

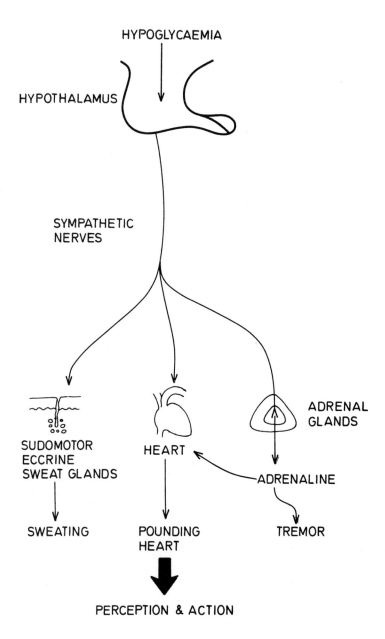

Figure 1. Autonomic activation and sympathetic neural stimulation of representative end-organs associated with common autonomic symptoms of hypoglycaemia.

of energy therefore renders it exceptionally vulnerable to hypoglycaemia and a fall in blood glucose reduces the delivery of glucose to the brain. The deprivation of glucose affects neuronal activity, causing abnormal cognitive function and information processing, which produces the development of neuroglycopenic symptoms. These include difficulty in concentrating, confusion, drowsiness, tiredness, and dizziness. A fall in the blood glucose below the normal range is detected within the central nervous system. To counteract this threat to the integrity of cerebral function, the autonomic centres in the hypothalamus are activated to stimulate the parasympathetic and sympathetic nervous systems. Sympathetic stimulation of various end-organs increases sudomotor gland activity to produce sweating (Corrall *et al.*, 1983), stimulates the heart to increase heart rate, myocardial contractility and cardiac output (Fisher *et al.*, 1987), and promotes the secretion of adrenaline from the adrenal medullary glands (Cannon *et al.*, 1924) (Figure 1). Hypoglycaemia is one of the most potent stimuli to provoke secretion of adrenaline (Cryer, 1980). Sympathetic activation causes noradrenaline to be secreted as a neurotransmitter, and despite a substantial quantity being reabsorbed into sympathetic nerve endings, a proportion enters the systemic circulation and can be measured in plasma.

The common autonomic symptoms are sweating, anxiety, tremor, palpitations, and a sensation of warmth (via vasodilatation). The increase in circulating plasma adrenaline promotes the development of tremor and augments the magnitude and possibly the perception of some of the autonomic symptoms. The autonomic symptoms are of primary importance in alerting an individual to the development of hypoglycaemia, although some diabetic patients, particularly those who have had diabetes for several years, may use neuroglycopenic symptoms to identify the development of a low blood glucose. However, the neuroglycopenic symptoms are inherently less reliable as the perception of symptoms may be impaired by neuroglycopenia per se.

Hormonal Responses to Acute Hypoglycaemia

The activation of the autonomic centres within the hypothalamus occurs concurrently with stimulation of secretion of various hypothalamic and pituitary hormones, some of which have a counterregulatory role (vasopressin, growth hormone, and adrenocorticotrophin), producing a rise in blood glucose. Other hormones are simultaneously released (prolactin and oxytocin) for which no physiological role in the modulation of blood glucose homeostasis has yet been identified. Hypoglycaemia also stimulates the secretion of glucagon from the alpha cells of the pancreatic islets, and this is the most effective of the counterregulatory hormones in promoting recovery of blood glucose (Cryer, 1981).

Awareness of Hypoglycaemia

Awareness of hypoglycaemia involves the perception and recognition of the onset of identifiable symptoms of hypoglycaemia. Previous experience of hypoglycaemia is important as there are wide individual or idiosyncratic differences in symptomatology and patients have to learn to recognise the constellation of symptoms which is peculiar to themselves. Symptoms which cause physiological manifestations can be easily identified by the subject, eg. sweating, palpitations (or pounding heart) and trembling, but neuroglycopenic symptoms are equally common at the time of initial perception of acute hypoglycaemia and may contribute to early awareness of hypoglycaemia (Hepburn et al., 1989a). Other non-physiological factors such as the time of day, the proximity to meal times (many diabetic patients experience hypoglycaemia before meals), the relationship to strenuous or unplanned exercise, and personal knowledge about preceding experience of susceptibility to hypoglycaemia also provide external cues to assist recognition of the onset of hypoglycaemia. This phase of awareness of hypoglycaemia may be relatively transient if the prevailing blood glucose does not continue to fall or is maintained experimentally at a constant level, because cerebral adaptation to neuroglycopenia occurs during moderate hypoglycaemia (Kerr et al., 1989). However, in everyday experience, insulin-treated patients with diabetes usually act upon their initial awareness of hypoglycaemia and take appropriate avoiding action by ingesting oral carbohydrate.

Historical and Clinical Background

From the time of the earliest clinical use of insulin to treat diabetes it has been recognised that some patients are unable to recognise the onset of hypoglycaemia and may proceed rapidly to hypoglycaemic coma (Banting et al., 1923; Baldimos and Root, 1959; Sussman et al., 1963). This problem of "hypoglycaemia unawareness" has usually been attributed to autonomic neuropathy (Hoeldtke et al., 1982), a complication of diabetes of long duration in which autonomic innervation is disrupted, and the usual activation of end organs does not occur. However, hypoglycaemia unawareness also affects patients who have no discernible objective evidence of peripheral autonomic dysfunction as assessed by conventional testing (Hepburn et al., 1990). The cause of this loss of symptomatic awareness in non-neuropathic patients is unclear, but in the chronic form it appears to be an acquired defect which occurs predominantly in patients who have had diabetes for more than ten years. Improvement of blood glucose control by intensification of insulin therapy also diminishes the perception of hypoglycaemic warning symptoms (Lager et al., 1986; Amiel et al., 1987), but this acute form is reversible.

Definition of Hypoglycaemia Awareness

We have proposed that awareness of hypoglycaemia can be classified on historical grounds into three categories:

1. Patients who are always aware of the onset of their hypoglycaemic episodes have *normal awareness*.
2. Patients who are aware of some but not all episodes of hypoglycaemia, or who have lost some but not all of their autonomic warning symptoms have *partial awareness*.
3. Patients who are unable to recognise the onset of hypoglycaemia at any time and may require external assistance to treat hypoglycaemia, have *absent awareness*.

To be included in either the *partial* or *absent* categories we have suggested that diabetic patients must give a consistent clinical history of this problem for at least one year, during which at least two documented episodes of hypoglycaemia have occurred (Hepburn et al., 1989b).

Human Insulin and Awareness of Hypoglycamia

For 60 years patients with diabetes were treated with animal insulins, extracted either from the pancreas of pigs (porcine insulin) or from cows (bovine insulin). Allergic reactions to these unpurified animal insulins were common, until refinement of production techniques introduced highly purified monocomponent insulins which almost eliminated allergic responses to animal insulins. Porcine and bovine insulins differ from human insulin by minor differences in amino acid sequences: porcine insulin differs by one amino acid and bovine insulin by three amino acids. Human insulin is now produced commercially by genetic engineering using recombinant DNA technology, and these preparations are highly purified and have minimal antigenicity (Fineberg et al., 1982). In the early 1980's, human insulin formulations were introduced for the routine treatment of patients with diabetes. In 1985–6 only about 6% of the insulin prescribed in the UK was of the human species (Pickup, 1986) but now at least three quarters of the 200,000 or so insulin-treated diabetic patients in the UK are using commercially produced human insulin (Pickup, 1989). Most patients with insulin-treated diabetes have been transferred without difficulty from insulins of animal origin to human insulin. Within the last two years, with increasing numbers of diabetic patients in European countries being transferred to human insulin, reports have appeared of adverse effects in some diabetic patients, in whom the transfer from animal to human insulin has been associated with a reduction in awareness of the onset of hypoglycaemia, coincidental with an alleged increase in the frequency of hypoglycaemia (Teuscher and Berger, 1987; Berger et al., 1989). These claims have been challenged by others (Berger, 1987; Gale, 1989).

Hypoglycaemia Unawareness and Human Insulin

The attenuation of symptoms of hypoglycaemia which has been tenuously associated with transfer to the human species of insulin has engendered much concern among long-standing insulin-treated diabetic patients, but it has not been described in new diabetic patients following treatment with human insulin. In Switzerland Teuscher and Berger (1987) have claimed that this problem of reduced awareness of hypoglycaemia affected one third of all diabetic patients who had been transferred from animal to human insulin, but surveys in Scotland have suggested a much smaller percentage (6–8%) of diabetic patients may be affected (Hepburn et al., 1989b; Duncan et al., 1990). Some of these patients may have developed preceding unawareness of hypoglycaemia as part of the natural history of diabetes and such patients were not excluded in the Swiss survey thus influencing the total number of affected patients. Improvement in glycaemic control or reduction in insulin antibodies may be other possible aetiological factors in causing this apparent change in hypoglycaemic symptoms. A subsequent study in Switzerland (Berger et al., 1989) which claimed to show a shift from autonomic to neuroglycopenic symptoms on human insulin, has been criticised with respect to the inappropriate allocation of symptoms to the autonomic and neuroglycopenic groups. It is therefore extremely important for the safety of diabetic patients that technology is developed which will allow objective estimation and quantification of any possible symptomatic or physiological differences in the manifestations of hypoglycaemia which may arise from the use of newly developed insulins.

We have used different methods to estimate and identify the subjective awareness of hypoglycaemia in diabetic patients, the nature and intensity of the symptoms which occur during acute hypoglycaemia and to obtain objective evidence of the onset of the autonomic activation which causes the development of autonomic warning symptoms.

Techniques for Assessment

Autonomic Activation

When investigating perception of the onset of hypoglycaemia in patients with diabetes it is valuable to provide objective evidence that autonomic activation has occurred (the autonomic REACTION) and to identify precisely its time of onset. When the autonomic neural discharge stimulates end organs, central feedback permits perception of the autonomic symptoms by the individual. Various tests can be used to assess the integrity of the autonomic nervous system, some of which are used routinely in clinical practice. These include cardiovascular autonomic reflexes, pupillary responses to light and tests of gastrointestinal motility (Ewing and Clarke, 1986). However, these are static investigations which provide information about the integrity of components and not about dynamic changes in the functioning of the autonomic nervous system over a short time period in response to a particular stimulus or stress. Fagius *et al.* (1986) have used microneurography, inserting a micro-electrode into a nerve to record muscle nerve sympathetic activity during hypoglycaemia, but this is a difficult and highly specialised technique which requires considerable expertise, and is impractical for routine use and is uncomfortable for the subject.

We have used two main types of dynamic indicators of the development of autonomic activation during hypoglycaemia; (a) hormonal and (b) physiological. The adrenal and pancreatic hormonal responses to hypoglycaemia, which we have designated as the *hormonal indicators* provide direct indices of autonomic activity, while hypothalamic-pituitary hormonal responses infer activity indirectly. The acute changes in the rate of sweating and of heart rate during hypoglycaemia, which we have designated as the *physiological indicators*, indicate a direct end-organ response to the central activation of autonomic centres.

Hormonal indicators

Pancreatic hormones   In addition to the combined sympathetic and parasympathetic neural discharge during acute insulin-induced hypoglycaemia there is simultaneous activation of a hypothalamic-pituitary hormonal response which is slower to manifest peripherally. One effect of parasympathetic neural stimulation is to cause the secretion of the hormone, pancreatic polypeptide, from the pancreatic islets which can be measured in the peripheral circulation by radioimmunoassay. While pancreatic polypeptide has no recognised role in the production of the autonomic warning symptoms, its secretion during hypoglycaemia is mediated entirely by parasympathetic cholinergic innervation via the vagus nerve (Schwartz *et al.*, 1978) and an obtunded increase in plasma pancreatic polypeptide in response to acute insulin-induced hypoglycaemia has been shown to be a sensitive and subtle indicator of the presence of early, and clinically undetectable, autonomic neuropathy (Krarup *et al.*, 1979; Kennedy *et al.*, 1988). The plasma pancreatic polypeptide response to hypoglycaemia can therefore be used as a qualitative indicator of activation of the autonomic nervous system, though it does not indicate the time of onset nor the intensity of the autonomic reaction.

Plasma catecholamines   A significant rise in plasma concentrations of adrenaline and noradrenaline occurs during acute insulin-induced hypoglycaemia and the maximum plasma concentrations achieved have been used as a measure of the magnitude or intensity of the autonomic activation which has occurred (Christensen, 1979). However, disruption or dysfunction of the peripheral autonomic nervous system also results in an obtunded rise in the plasma concentration of these hormones, particularly adrenaline (Hoeldtke *et al.*, 1982). In tetraplegic subjects, in whom the sympathetic outflow is completely disrupted by transection of the cervical sympathetic chain, neither plasma adrenaline nor plasma noradrenaline rise in response to hypoglycaemia (Palmer *et al.*, 1976; Corrall *et al.*, 1979; Mathias *et al.*, 1979). Although the magnitude of the catecholamine response is a useful index of autonomic stimulation, the maximal plasma concentration does not occur until 15 minutes after induction of the acute autonomic reaction by insulin infusion (Fisher *et al.*, 1987; Frier *et al.*, 1988) so that plasma measurements do not provide a rapid indicator of the onset of autonomic secretion.

Hypothalamo-pituitary hormones   Acute insulin-induced hypoglycaemia has been used for many years to test the integrity of hypothalamic-anterior pituitary function, stimulating the release of growth hormone, prolactin and adrenocorticotrophin (ACTH) from the anterior pituitary gland, and the subsequent secretion of cortisol from the adrenal cortex. The opioid peptide, beta-endorphin, is released in parallel with ACTH, with which it shares a common precursor from the pituitary gland (Bright *et al.*, 1983). The hypothalamus is the other major site of synthesis of beta-endorphin within the central nervous system, and beta-endorphin has a role in the hypothalamic-pituitary response to stress. Simultaneous release of vasopressin (Baylis *et al.*, 1981) and oxytocin (Fisher *et al.*, 1989) occurs via the posterior pituitary gland. The rise in the plasma concentrations of all of these hormones can be used to assess the integrity of the hypothalamic-pituitary response, and hence indicate indirectly the timing of stimulation of the hypothalamic autonomic centres in response to acute insulin-induced hypoglycaemia (Frier *et al.*, 1988).

The major drawback in using these hypothalamic-pituitary hormones to indicate the timing of onset of autonomic activation is the delay in demonstrating their secretion, as most hormones do not reach a maximal plasma concentration until fifteen minutes or more after the onset of the acute autonomic reaction has been detected by physiological tests. All of these hormones require laboratory estimation, some of which require specialist assay expertise and expensive reagents. These limitations therefore exclude hormonal indicators as measurements which can be used to identify the time of the acute onset of autonomic activation and limit their value to demonstrating putative central hypothalamic dysfunction in which pituitary dysfunction has been postulated to occur in parallel with a reduction in autonomic activation (Frier *et al.*, 1988). An obtunded rise in adrenaline, noradrenaline and pancreatic polypeptide may result either from central autonomic dysfunction or from damage to the peripheral autonomic nerves, and their use as indicators of the activation of hypothalamic autonomic centres may be open to variable interpretation in diabetic patients who have established microvascular and neuropathic complications.

Physiological indicators

Haemodynamic indicators In attempting to overcome the limitations of using hormonal indicators to identify the onset of autonomic activation we have examined dynamic measurements of autonomic stimulation which occur during acute hypoglycaemia. The profound haemodynamic changes of hypoglycaemia include a rapid rise in heart rate and changes in blood pressure with a rise in systolic, a fall in diastolic and no change in mean arterial blood pressure (Christensen *et al.*, 1979). The rapid increase in heart rate is easily recorded using precordial electrocardiogram leads, occurs before the change in blood pressure and is temporally distinct from the maximal rise in plasma adrenaline concentration. It is therefore a suitable dynamic cardiovascular indicator of the acute autonomic activation.

Perspiration monitors We have refined an earlier technique (Corrall *et al.*, 1983) to effect a dynamic and continuous measurement of the rate of sweat production during hypoglycaemia. Using a sampling capsule attached to an area of skin, usually on the anterior abdominal wall, dry gas is blown across the skin at a steady rate, and the sweat produced is evaporated and passed to a hygrometer. This measures humidity, thereby providing a continuous record of the sweat produced. An example of a recording of sweat production during hypoglycaemia in a normal healthy subject is demonstrated in figure 2, the rapid rise in humidity of the ventilated gas indicating an increase in sweat production. In a previous study (Corrall *et al.*, 1983) the onset of sweating coincided with the acute autonomic reaction, and in our own observations the sweating response occurred when blood glucose had declined to a specific concentration during the induction of acute hypoglycaemia; at that threshold a sudden and rapid increase in the rate of sweating was observed. Thereafter a plateau was reached and during blood glucose recovery the rate of sweating gradually fell until the basal rate of sweating was restored. Although the duration of sweating depended upon the duration of hypoglycaemia it also varied greatly between individuals despite exposure to a similar degree of hypoglycaemia, as shown previously (Corrall *et al.*, 1983). However, the onset of the rapid increase in sweating coincided very closely with the onset of the rapid rise in heart rate during acute hypoglycaemia and the two parameters can therefore be used to identify the onset of the acute autonomic neural discharge. Both of these indices may be affected by peripheral autonomic dysfunction so that the responses in patients with severe autonomic neuropathy may be obtunded. Sweating does not occur in response to hypoglycaemia in sympathectomized subjects (Frier, 1981), and is apparently exaggerated in patients taking beta-blocking drugs, although this has not been estimated objectively (Clausen-Sjobom *et al.*, 1987).

Tremor measurements In addition to the indicators which have been described to identify the onset of the autonomic activation, the amplitude of tremor during hypoglycaemia can be measured using an accelerometer placed on a finger. Tremor is stimulated by adrenaline and the amplitude of tremor correlates closely with the magnitude of the prevailing plasma adrenaline concentration (Fellows *et al.*, 1986). The amplitude of tremor was used to assess the degree of adrenergic stimulation at different levels of hypoglycaemia induced by a glucose/insulin clamp technique, although with this experimental technique the degree, but not the onset of sympatho-adrenal stimulation is measured (*Heller et al.*, 1987). Finger tremor could presumably be monitored continuously throughout the induction of hypoglycaemia and so be used to identify the onset of an objective increase in tremor amplitude. However, because of the close relationship between tremor and the ambient or circulating plasma adrenaline, a significant increase in tremor amplitude may not occur until after the acute onset of autonomic activation when plasma adrenaline concentration rises significantly. In this respect the previously described physiological indicators may have greater sensitivity to identify the acute onset of the autonomic response, but the onset of tremor has not been studied during induction of acute hypoglycaemia.

Neuroglycopenia and Cognitive Dysfunction

Cognitive function tests

Cerebral glucopenia during acute hypoglycaemia causes dysfunction of neuronal activity. Unlike immutable structural derangements, hypoglycaemia-related neuropsychological deficits appear to be reversible with restoration of the blood glucose to normal. Studies have documented slowness of reasoning, memory, and fine motor skills during insulin-induced hypoglycaemia when compared to normoglycaemia (Holmes *et al.*, 1983; Pramming *et al.*, 1986; Stevens *et al.*, 1989). A variety of cognitive function tests have since been used to assess cognitive dysfunction and include: choice reaction time, visual reaction time, trail-making tests A and B, and digit span tests (Herold *et al.*, 1985; Holmes *et al.*, 1986; Heller *et al.*, 1987; Hoffman *et al.*, 1989; Stevens *et al.*, 1989). Some of these cognitive function tests which involve sensory input, central processing and motor coordination, such as choice reaction time and trail-making test B, have proved to be sensitive in identifying subtle cognitive dysfunction during hypoglycaemia (Stevens *et al.*, 1989). These bedside tests are able to identify neuroglycopenia at blood glucose concentrations above the level at which autonomic activation develops and subjective symptoms commence. However, because each test takes a finite time to process they can only be applied at intervals during hypoglycaemia and therefore cannot effectively identify dynamic changes in cognitive functioning during acute hypoglycaemia. Also some of these tests such as the trail-making tests are subject to practice effects which may make them more difficult to interpret.

Neurophysiological tests

In an attempt to identify more subtle changes in cognitive function which may precede the onset of the autonomic activation and the development of hypoglycaemic symptoms, some workers have utilised central neurophysiological investigations, which include visually evoked responses, continuous electroencephalography and brainstem evoked responses to monitor p300 latency measurements (Harrad *et al.*, 1985; De Feo *et al.*, 1988; Pramming *et al.*, 1988; Tamburrano *et al.*, 1988; Blackman *et al*, 1990). Although these techniques are potentially able to demonstrate very early changes in neuronal functioning during the initial decline in blood glucose, this methodology is not applicable to dynamic measurement and does not continuously measure neurological function. Some authors have attempted to use continuously recorded electroencephalogram (EEG) tracings to detect neurological dysfunction during acute hypoglycaemia, but have encountered various difficulties. Some studies have shown definitive EEG changes (development of delta waves) only at very low blood glucose concentrations which did not correlate with the development of hypoglycaemic symptoms (S. A. Amiel, personal communication). In addition neuroglycopenia sometimes induces somnolence, so that the subject may fall asleep during the study. Sleep can result in pronounced EEG changes which may be confused with the EEG changes provoked by hypoglycaemia. No ideal dynamic and continuous technique is yet available to monitor neuronal function and identify the precise onset of cognitive dysfunction.

Symptoms of Hypoglycaemia

The autonomic warning symptoms can be used to identify the onset of acute autonomic activation. The frequency and intensity of symptoms can be recorded throughout hypoglycaemia by administering a symptom questionnaire at regular intervals and by using a scoring system; the time of onset of symptoms and variations in their magnitude can also be assessed. This permits the hierarchy of symptoms, both autonomic and neuroglycopenic, to be identified and alerts the subject to the onset of hypoglycaemia. However, the role of the individual in reporting the onset of their own symptoms introduces considerable subjectivity to this measurement and in those diabetic patients who have unawareness of hypoglycaemia it may be of no value as they are unable to rely on the development of autonomic symptoms to detect hypoglycaemia. This suggestion has been supported by some of our recent studies investigating diabetic patients who had lost their awareness of the onset of hypoglycaemia, but who had no objective evidence of coexisting autonomic neuropathy. These patients were unable to report any warning symptoms before severe hypoglycaemia developed during which they became significantly and overtly neuroglycopenic. However, following the development of neuroglycopenia, the objective physiological indicators of autonomic activation (rise in heart rate and rapid increase in sweating) were

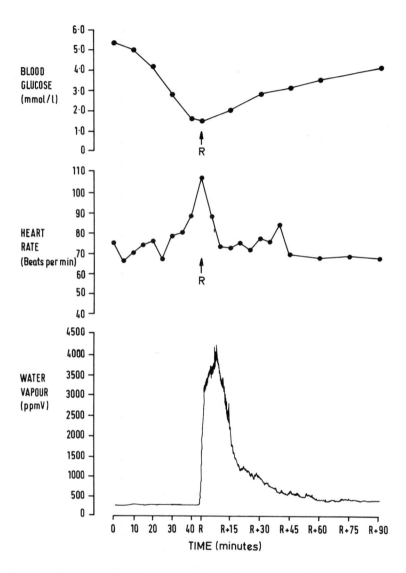

Figure 2. The individual heart rate and sweating responses from a normal (non-diabetic) human subject during acute insulin-induced hypoglycaemia. Blood glucose is demonstrated in the upper panel, heart rate in the middle panel and sweat production, expressed as ppmV of water vapour, in the lower panel. The increase in sweat production and rise in heart rate occurs very rapidly and coincided in the non-diabetic individuals with the nadir of blood glucose and the acute autonomic reaction (R).

identified and indicated the presence of an acute autonomic reaction and the lower blood glucose concentration required to trigger this response, despite the patients' subjective inability to perceive the onset of hypoglycaemia (Hepburn *et al.*, 1989c). The acute neuroglycopenia in these patients with hypoglycaemia unawareness impaired their ability to perceive the warning autonomic symptoms. The hormonal indicators were also used in these studies to confirm retrospectively the occurrence and the magnitude of the autonomic response to acute hypoglycaemia.

Conclusions

In conclusion, there are problems inherent in using purely patient-based reporting to identify acute autonomic activation and the accompanying symptoms. This is related to the subjective nature of such measurements, particularly in individuals who have developed unawareness of hypoglycaemia. New technology has enabled the use of objective physio-logical indicators supported by the retrospective measurement of hormonal indicators, to effectively identify the onset and the magnitude of the autonomic activation in individual subjects. Neuroglycopenia, which may interfere with perception of the autonomic warning symptoms, can also be assessed in a practical manner using a variety of neuropsychological tests, although no ideal test is yet available which can be applied continuously throughout experimental hypoglycaemia with either varying or static blood glucose concentrations. These simple objective tests can now be used during investigations of awareness and perception of hypoglycaemia and may prove useful in the investigation of any possible differences in symptoms of hypoglycaemia in diabetic patients converted to any newly developed insulin types. They are essential during studies which seek to identify and quantitate potential differences in awareness and symptomatology which may be ascribed to the use of different insulin species or formulations or when hypoglycaemia is induced by different methods in which factors such as the rate of fall of blood glucose are variable.

References

Amiel S.A., Tamborlane W.V., Simonson D.C. and Sherwin R.S. (1987). Defective glucose counterregulation after strict glycemic control of insulin-dependent diabetes mellitus. *New England Journal of Medicine* **316**, 1376–1383.

Baldimos M.C. and Root H.F. (1959). Hypoglycemic insulin reactions without warning symptoms. *Journal of the American Medical Association* **171**, 261–266.

Banting F.G., Campbell W.R. and Fletcher A.A. (1923). Further clinical experience with insulin (pancreatic extracts) in the treatment of diabetes mellitus. *British Medical Journal*, 8–12.

Baylis P.H., Zerbe R.L. and Robertson G.L. (1981). Arginine vasopressin response to insulin-induced hypoglycemia in man. *Journal of Clinical Endocrinology and Metabolism* 53, 935–940.

Berger M. (1987). Human insulin: much ado about hypoglycaemia (un)awareness. *Diabetologia* 30, 829–833.

Berger W.G., Keller U., Honegger B. and Jaeggi E. (1989). Warning symptoms of hypoglycaemia during treatment with human and porcine insulin in diabetes mellitus. *Lancet* i, 1041–1044.

Blackman J.D., Towle V.L., Lewis G.F., Spire J. and Polonsky K.S. (1990). Hypoglycemic thresholds for cognitive dysfunction in humans. *Diabetes* 39, 828–835.

Bright G.M., Kaiser D.L., Rogol A.D. and Clarke W.L. (1983). Naloxone attenuates recovery from insulin-induced hypoglycemia in normal man. *Journal of Clinical Endocrinology and Metabolism* 57, 213–216.

Cannon W.B., McIver M.A. and Bliss S.W. (1924). Studies on the conditions of activity in endocrine glands. XIII A sympathetic and adrenal mechanism for mobilising sugar in hypoglycemia. *American Journal of Physiology* 69, 46–66.

Christensen N.J. (1979). Catecholamines in diabetes mellitus. *Diabetologia* 16, 211–264.

Clausen-Sjobom N., Lins P.E., Adamson U., Curstedt T. and Hamberger B. (1987). Effects of metoprolol on the counter-regulation and recognition of prolonged hypoglycemia in insulin-dependent diabetics. *Acta Medica Scandinavica* 222, 57–63.

Corrall R.J.M., Frier B.M., McClemont E.J.W., Taylor S.J. and Christie N.E. (1979). Recovery mechanisms from acute hypoglycaemia in complete tetraplegia. *Paraplegia* 17, 314–318.

Corrall R.J.M., Frier B.M., Davidson N.McD., Hopkins W.M. and French E.B. (1983). Cholinergic manifestations of the acute autonomic reaction to hypoglycaemia in man. *Clinical Science* 64, 49–53.

Cryer P.E. (1980). Physiology and pathophysiology of the human sympathoadrenal neuroendocrine system. *New England Journal of Medicine* 303, 436–444.

Cryer P.E. (1981). Glucose counterregulation in man. *Diabetes* 30, 261–264.

De Feo P., Gallai V., Mazzotta G., Crispino G., Torlone E., Perriello G., *et al.* (1988). Modest decrements in plasma glucose concentration cause early impairment in cognitive function and later activation of glucose counterregulation in the absence of hypoglycemic symptoms in normal man. *Journal of Clinical Investigation* 82, 436–444.

Duncan C., Campbell I.W., McBain A.M. and Jones I.G. (1990). Hypoglycaemia survey in insulin-dependent diabetic population at time of change from beef to human insulin. *Practical Diabetes* 7, 18–19.

Ewing D.J. and Clarke B.F. (1986). Diabetic autonomic neuropathy: present insights and future prospects. *Diabetes Care* 9, 648–665.

Fagius J., Niklasson F. and Berne C. (1986). Sympathetic outflow in human muscle nerves increases during hypoglycemia. *Diabetes* 35, 1124–1129.

Fellows I.W., MacDonald I.A., Wharrad H.J. and Birmingham A.T. (1986). Low plasma concentrations of adrenaline and physiological tremor in man. *Journal of Neurology, Neurosurgery and Psychiatry* 49, 296–399.

Fineberg S.E., Galloway J.A., Fineberg N.S. and Rathbun M.J. (1982). Immunologic improvement resulting from the transfer of animal insulin-treated diabetic subjects to human insulin (recombinant DNA). *Diabetes Care* 5 (Suppl 2), 107–113.

Fisher B.M., Gillen G., Dargie H.J., Inglis G.C. and Frier B.M. (1987). The effects of insulin-induced hypoglycaemia on cardiovascular function in normal man: studies using radionuclide ventriculography. *Diabetologia* **30**, 841–845.

Fisher B.M., Baylis P.H., Thornton S. and Frier B.M. (1989). Arginine vasopressin and oxytocin responses to insulin-induced hypoglycemia in type 1 (insulin-dependent) diabetes. *Journal of Clinical Endocrinology and Metabolism* **68**, 688–692.

Frier B.M. (1981) MD Thesis. Acute hypoglycaemia in man. University of Edinburgh.

Frier B.M. (1986). Hypoglycaemia and diabetes. *Diabetic Medicine* **3**, 513–525.

Frier B.M., Fisher B.M., Gray C.E. and Beastall G.H. (1988). Counterregulatory hormonal responses to hypoglycaemia in type 1 (insulin-dependent) diabetes: evidence for diminished hypothalamic-pituitary hormonal secretion. *Diabetologia* **31**, 421–429.

Gale E.A.M. (1989). Hypoglycaemia and human insulin. *Lancet* **ii**, 1264–1266.

Harrad R.A., Cockram C.S., Plumb A.P., Stone S., Fenwick P. and Sonksen P.H. (1985). The effect of hypoglycaemia on visual function: a clinical and electrophysiological study. *Clinical Science* **69**, 673–679.

Heller S.R., MacDonald I.A., Herbert M. and Tattersall R.B. (1987). Influence of sympathetic nervous system on hypoglycaemic warning symptoms. *Lancet* **ii**, 359–363.

Hepburn D.A., Fisher B.M., Patrick A.W. and Frier B.M. (1989a) Neuroglycopenic symptoms are commonly associated with the onset of awareness of hypoglycaemia in normal and type 1 diabetic subjects. *Diabetic Medicine* **6** (Suppl 2), 32A.

Hepburn D.A., Eadington D.W., Patrick A.W., Colledge N.R. and Frier B.M. (1989b). Symptomatic awareness of hypoglycaemia: does it change on transfer from animal to human insulin? *Diabetic Medicine* **6**,586–590.

Hepburn D.A., Patrick A.W. and Frier B.M. (1989c). Severe neuroglycopenia precedes autonomic activation during acute insulin-induced hypoglycemia in insulin-dependent diabetic patients with hypoglycemic unawareness. *Diabetes* **38** (Suppl 2), 76A.

Hepburn D.A., Patrick A.W., Eadington D.W., Ewing D.J. and Frier B.M. (1990). Unawareness of hypoglycaemia in insulin-treated diabetic patients: prevalence and relationship to autonomic neuropathy. *Diabetic Medicine* **7**, 711–717.

Herold K.C., Polonsky K.S., Cohen R.M., Levy J. and Douglas F. (1985). Variable deterioration in cortical function during insulin-induced hypoglycaemia. *Diabetes* **34**, 677–685.

Hoeldtke R.D., Boden G., Shuman C.R. and Owen O.E. (1982). Reduced epinephrine secretion and hypoglycemia unawareness in diabetic autonomic neuropathy. *Annals of Internal Medicine* **96**, 459–462.

Hoffman R.G., Speelman D.J., Hinnen D.A., Conley K.L., Guthrie R.A. and Knapp R.K. (1989). Changes in cortical functioning with acute hypoglycemia and hyperglycemia in type 1 diabetes. *Diabetes Care* **12**, 193–197.

Holmes C.S., Hayford J.T., Gonzalez J.L. and Weydert J.A. (1983). A survey of cognitive functioning at different blood glucose levels in diabetic persons. *Diabetes Care* **6**, 180–185.

Holmes C.S., Koepe K.M. and Thompson R.G. (1986). Simple versus complex performance impairments at three blood glucose levels. *Psychoneuroendocrinology* **11**, 353–357.

Kennedy F.P., Go V.L.W., Cryer P.E., Bolli G.B. and Gerich J.E. (1988) Subnormal pancreatic polypeptide and epinephrine responses to insulin-induced hypoglycemia identify patients with insulin-dependent diabetes mellitus predisposed to develop overt autonomic neuropathy. *Annals International Medicine* **108**, 54–58.

Kerr D., MacDonald I.A. and Tattersall R.B. (1989). Adaptation to mild hypoglycaemia in normal subjects despite sustained increases in counter-regulatory hormones. *Diabetologia* **32**, 249–254.

Krarup T., Schwartz T.W., Hilsted J., Madsbad S., Verlaege O. and Sestoft L. (1979). Impaired response of pancreatic polypeptide to hypoglycaemia: an early sign of autonomic neuropathy in diabetics. *British Medical Journal* **2**, 1544–1546.

Lager I., Attvall S., Blohme G. and Smith U. (1986). Altered recognition of hypoglycaemic symptoms in type 1 diabetes during intensified control with continuous subcutaneous insulin infusion. *Diabetic Medicine* **3**, 322–325.

Mathias C.J., Frankel J.L., Turner R.C. and Christensen N.J. (1979). Physiological responses to insulin hypoglycaemia in spinal man. *Paraplegia* **17**, 319–326.

Palmer J.P., Henry D.P., Benson J.W., Johnson D.G. and Ensinck J.W. (1976). Glucagon responses to hypoglycemia in sympathectomized man. *Journal Clinical Investigation* **57**, 522–525.

Pickup J.C. (1986). Human insulin. *British Medical Journal* **292**, 155–157.

Pickup J.C. (1989). Human insulin. Problems with hypoglycaemia in a few patients. *British Medical Journal* **299**, 991–993.

Pramming S., Thorsteinsson B., Theilgaard A., Pinner E.M. and Binder C. (1986). Cognitive function during hypoglycaemia in type 1 diabetes mellitus. *British Medical Journal* **292**, 647–650.

Pramming S., Thorsteinsson B., Stigsby B. and Binder C. (1988). Glycaemic threshold for changes in electroencephalograms during hypoglycaemia in patients with insulin dependent diabetes. *British Medical Journal* **296**, 665–667.

Schwartz T.W., Holst J.J., Fahrenkrug J., Lindkaer-Jensen S., Neilsen O.V. *et al.* (1978). Vagal cholinergic regulation of pancreatic polypeptide secretion. *Journal of Clinical Investigation* **61**, 781–789.

Stevens A.B., McKane W.R., Bell P.M., Bell P., King D.J. and Hayes J.R. (1989). Psychomotor performance and counterregulatory responses during mild hypoglycemia in healthy volunteers. *Diabetes Care* **12**, 12–17.

Sussman K.E., Crout J.R. and Marble A. (1963). Failure of warning in insulin-induced hypoglycemic reactions. *Diabetes* **12**, 38–45.

Tamburrano G., Lala A., Locuratolo N., Leonetti F., Sbraccia P., Giaccari A., *et al.* (1988). Electroencephalography and visually evoked potentials during moderate hypoglycemia. *Journal of Clinical Endocrinology and Metabolism* **66**, 1301–1306.

Teuscher A. and Berger W.G. (1987). Hypoglycaemia unawareness in diabetics transferred from beef/porcine insulin to human insulin. *Lancet* **ii**, 382–385.

The DCCT Research Group. (1987). Diabetes control and complications trial (DCCT): results of feasibility study. *Diabetes Care* **10**, 1–19.

Implantable Insulin Infusion Pumps in the Management of Diabetes

Philip Home

Freeman Diabetes Unit, University of Newcastle upon Tyne, UK.

Introduction

Insulin delivery in people who do not have diabetes is sophisticated and refined. Quite why evolution should have been driven to achieve this remains unclear, but it can be speculated that the answer lies in the control of blood glucose concentrations, the major, although not the only biochemical substance regulated by insulin. The physiological concentration of glucose in blood and tissue fluids is very tightly limited, perhaps because glucose although essential to life, is also toxic in higher concentrations to cell membranes and in particular to vascular endothelium. This may be the cause of the widespread vascular damage in people with diabetes, which in turn leads to the catastrophic later complications of diabetes.

This tight control of blood glucose levels by insulin is achieved through a series of mechanisms. Firstly blood glucose concentrations are continuously sensed by the islet B-cells that produce insulin, and the signal from these glucose concentrations is used to modulate the secretion and synthesis of insulin. Secondly other information affecting glucose metabolism, such as eating or exercise, is also conveyed to the islet B-cell, and similarly used to modulate insulin secretion. Finally, insulin secretion is itself a continuous process, with regulation occurring on a minute to minute basis, so that fine tuning of insulin delivery can be achieved.

All this is in contrast to the insulin delivery used in insulin-requiring diabetes. As insulin is a protein and therefore cannot be taken by mouth, it was inevitable in 1922 that it should be given by subcutaneous injection, as were many other drugs at that time. However insulin is absorbed only slowly into the blood from subcutaneous tissue, delivery cannot be finely controlled, and certainly not finely tuned to glucose concentrations or physiological needs. Furthermore since insulin delivery is then prospective, and not responsive to minute to minute changes in lifestyle, good blood glucose control can be achieved only by restrictions on the patient's behaviour, particularly in respect of eating. Added to this is the problem of erratic absorption of insulin from subcutaneous tissue, in particular giving rise to insulin concentrations which may be too high, with resulting hypoglycaemia. These problems would seem to account for much of the stress of having diabetes felt by the insulin-requiring patient, rather than the difficulty of self-administration of insulin itself, which appears to be relatively well tolerated by most patients.

A better insulin delivery system needs therefore to have certain characteristics, essentially in that it has to imitate some the properties of physiological insulin secretion:

1. In sensing glucose concentrations, a problem addressed by John Pickup in this book;
2. In being able to receive information about glucose levels, or other events such as the intention to eat or exercise;
3. In being able to change insulin delivery rate rapidly in response to such information;
4. In delivering that insulin into a site from which absorption into the blood is immediate, or at least consistent.

In the 1970s, when these problems were first seriously addressed, the received wisdom was that the glucose sensing and insulin delivery problems could be rapidly solved by intensive application of existing technology, but that the information handling would remain problematic because of the need for considerable computing power. In practice the opposite has turned out to be true, communications and computer technology having advanced beyond what could be anticipated, while glucose sensing or delivery of small quantities of insulin in the environment of the human body have proved difficult to achieve.

An approach to more physiological insulin delivery is to use an injection pump rather than a syringe, and to give the insulin directly into a vein rather than into subcutaneous tissue (Slama *et al.*, 1974). Indeed such an approach has been used for many years in hospitals, for example during surgery on diabetic patients, a situation when fine tuning of insulin delivery is even more important, and where considerable manpower is available to monitor glucose levels and adjust insulin delivery rates accordingly. During the 1970's and 1980's attempts were made to extend such technology to insulin delivery at home (Pickup *et al.*, 1980), but these ideas ran up against a series of problems:

1. Externally worn pumps are a physical and cosmetic inconvenience to many patients;
2. From an external pump an insulin delivery line (cannula) must cross the skin to the required delivery site. This provided a portal of entry for infection;
3. Insulin proved rather unstable in current preparations when kept at body temperature and agitated continually;
4. It proved difficult to find cannula materials that did not result in tissue reactions after long periods of insulin infusion into one site;

5. Some patients appeared to find it difficult to adjust to either handling a
    technological device, or being reminded of their diabetes by it, or being
    apparently dependent on it for health (Home and Marshall, 1984).

Because of these problems considerable effort has been put into the development of insulin delivery devices which lie within the body, just as a heart
pacemaker controls heart rate from a box under the skin. The present chapter is
concerned with the status and problems of such implantable insulin delivery
devices.

The Present Status of Implantable Insulin Pumps

In the early 1980's the only implantable pump available for insulin delivery
was a constant rate device (Kritz et al., 1983). The pump was driven by the
vapour pressure above a volatile liquid, a pressure which remains constant at
constant temperature. Unfortunately this also meant that the insulin delivery
rate was determined only by the concentration of insulin in the pump reservoir,
no allowance being possible for increased mealtime insulin requirements,
decreased requirements during exercise, or even changes in insulin sensitivity
from week to week. Furthermore the insulin-glycerol mixture used in the
pump gradually lost potency over a period of time, while in some cases insulin
precipitated in the cannula, causing the pump to slow down.

   Despite these problems constant rate pumps were used in fairly large
numbers in some centres (Irsigler et al., 1987), and proved the feasibility of
using such devices in diabetic patients, even under adverse circumstances.
Such pumps were never the subject of adequately controlled trials to assess
effectiveness when compared to external infusion devices, but uncontrolled
results suggested reasonably good blood glucose control despite the lack of
flexibility in insulin delivery. Formal investigation of patient acceptability
was never investigated, but appeared good, particularly as the lack of extra
mealtime insulin delivery meant supplementary injections were usually
necessary.

   The use of constant rate pumps did however highlight some other technical
problems of implantable devices, problems just as significant in considering
the second generation programmable devices:

1. By their very nature implantable devices have to placed within the body
    by a surgical procedure. Pacemakers are small enough to be placed below
    the clavicle, but an insulin pump, with its reservoir, pumping mechanism,
    and communications and control electronics, is considerably larger
    (presently 90 mm diameter, Table 1), and is usually placed in the deeper
    tissues of the anterior abdominal wall. The resulting scar is significant
    and permanent, and the device all too visible except in the very obese.
    Furthermore foreign bodies are prone to migrate within the tissues unless

strongly anchored, a particular problem with larger implantable devices. Surgical procedures carry risks, albeit small if the patient will tolerate a local anaesthetic, but more importantly infections can occur and are a problem when a foreign body is present in the tissues, and particularly in people with diabetes;

2. The devices have a finite life, and although in the constant rate devices this was generally related to insulin stability problems, in the newer devices the power source is usually a battery, at whose failure the entire pump needs to be replaced (Selam, 1988). Aside from the need to subject the patient to recurrent surgical procedures, the devices are expensive (second generation pumps around UK£8000) and likely to remain so;

3. Problems of biocompatibility remain. This is particularly true for the delivery cannulae, whose tips are generally placed either in the great veins or in the peritoneal cavity around the intestines. In both these sites the body has particularly active mechanisms for reacting to foreign materials, and in veins this can lead to thrombosis, while in the peritoneum fibrosis can lead to obstruction of insulin delivery.

Table 1   *Typical specification of an implantable insulin infusion pump*

Weight	200–300 g
Size	90 x 30 mm
Reservoir	10–25 ml
Battery life	> 3 yr

Nevertheless three manufacturers have developed and tested the more sophisticated programmable pumps, though experience in diabetic patients is as yet fairly limited. These devices are characterized by having the facility to deliver fluids at variable rates, according to preprogramming of the pump, and can thus give insulin according to what is judged to be future requirements, to cope with mealtimes, exercise, or even just variation in sensitivity to insulin between different times of the day. As the pump is implanted it is in effect remote from the user, and communication with the pump therefore has to be by telemetry across the skin, using a portable programmer. This of course has to be carried around by the patient, and sophisticated electronic safeguards need to be built into the systems to ensure that insulin delivery rate is not changed inadvertently by stray signals, interference, or programmer error.

The problems of insulin stability with the pump and pump cannula appear to have been solved by the development of surface active agents which protect the insulin molecule against chemical and physical stresses. Nevertheless it inevitably remains the case that the pump reservoir needs to be refilled at regular intervals, every 3 to 8 weeks depending on type. As this involves transgressing the skin, and hence a risk of introducing infection, and as it is important not to damage the pump or the entry port while refilling, the technique is a formal procedure carried out at the hospital. This will include exposure of the pump site, skin preparation with antiseptic solution, covering of surrounding areas with sterile towels, a local anaesthetic, and lying still for some minutes while the refill itself is performed.

Problems in the Use of Implantable Pumps

Problems in the use of implantable pumps are summarized in Table 2, and many are addressed above. It will be recognised that most of the major technical problems are now largely resolved, although major difficulties remain. Thus, while insulin stability and precipitation problems have not been reported with the new specially devised preparations, the long term safety of some of the required additives remains to be established, and absence of damage to pump mechanisms can really be established only over the lifetime of the pump in a large cohort of patients. Similarly the experience gained in the surgical placement of the earlier constant rate pumps has lead to a very significant decrease in local problems in the hands of experienced surgeons, but it is not known if this expertise can be generalized for more widespread use of these devices.

Table 2   *Problems encountered in the use of implantable insulin infusion pumps.*

Technical problems
 Catheter occlusion (insulin precipitates)
 Catheter obstruction (tissue reaction or thrombosis)
 Pump breakdown
 Surgical problems
  Wound infection
  Pump migration
 Need for refill at hospital

Patient problems
 Cosmetic problems
 Discomfort
 Use of programmer
  Empathy with technical devices
  Permanent companion
 Denial of diabetes

Cost of device and programmer

Reliability of these devices can be considered from two angles with differing impacts on the patient. Firstly overdosage of insulin can be fatal, either directly through unconsciousness due to severe hypoglycaemia, or indirectly through cognitive impairment during more mild hypoglycaemia. Pump stoppage can also be serious if the absence of insulin delivery goes undetected, as the patient can drift into ketoacidosis. Nevertheless insulin deficiency is fairly easily detected (through rising blood glucose levels), and the electronic checks built into these devices therefore stop the pump should an error be detected. This is analogous to demand heart pacemakers which default into a potentially dangerous fixed rate mode if their sensing systems no longer work, this mode being however more desirable than complete cessation of function. With programmable pumps detection of the error can be communicated to the user at the next time the programmer is used to change pump delivery rate, normally the next mealtime.

Secondly pump breakdown requires a surgical procedure for removal of the pump, and, at the time, decision as to whether to provide a replacement device at considerable cost. Fortunately the newer devices from two of the manufacturers have proved very reliable, and it appears that failure rates before exhaustion of planned battery life may be below 1%.

A difficulty that was encountered with external pumps can also be expected with implantable devices with further experience. Where blood glucose control becomes erratic in an individual for no apparent reason, the question is raised as to whether the pump is at fault. The medical approach to this problem is to check pump function using the programmed facilities provided, and to check insulin delivery by flushing the cannula, or even inspecting the cannula tip by direct or radiographic visualization. Even if no pump malfunction is detected experience suggests that a proportion of patients will remain convinced of intermittent device malfunction, apparently preferring that explanation to attributing the difficulty to some undetected medical or behavioural problem. In many cases this will lead to surgical removal of the expensive apparatus.

Other patient problems (Table 2) remain inadequately addressed by studies performed with implantable pumps to date, and certainly the long term cosmetic consequences of both the scarring and pump bulk are largely ignored by current investigators. The cosmetic problems are however likely to be of significance because:

1. Current pumps are large enough to distort skin contour, and thus affect the clothing that can be worn over them;
2. Modern society places considerable emphasis on perfection in bodily form and in holiday recreations which involve wearing very little clothing;
3. Much of the need for improved insulin delivery is in adolescents and young adults, the age group often most sensitive to body form and the need to conform to peer group behaviour patterns.

Experience from pacemakers is unhelpful in these respects, mainly because the overwhelming majority of these devices are used in the elderly, but also because they are smaller, and, in filling the infraclavicular fossa, much less obvious.

Discomfort is also little assessed as yet. This problem will not be easy to analyse, as complaints of chronic discomfort may really be a statement of lack of empathy with the system as a whole.

The third patient-related problem with implantable devices is concerned with the acceptability of technical devices for maintenance of health by some patients. The problem was never tackled properly with external devices, for many of those patients with a dislike of technical devices merely refused to take part in clinical trials, thus effectively biasing the study population. It might however be argued that such experience would anyway be irrelevant to implantable pumps, which in any case are not handled by the patient, and in many respects are 'invisible'. Nevertheless it is the case that to use programmable pumps the patient must use the external programmer, at least at every mealtime, and although these are easy to operate by those prepared to use a simple calculator-type keyboard, not every patient can be expected to handle these with empathy. Furthermore some confidence is needed that the pump is responding to the commands given (there is no visible or physical evidence of this), and although the external programmer will provide confirmation that the correct instruction has been received, lack of such confidence can be expected to lead to some anxiety in at least a small minority of patients.

An additional potential problem for patients, that might seem trivial at first sight, is the need to carry the external programmer with them nearly all the time, as it will be required whenever meals are taken. Presently these modules are not small, often 150 x 75 x 25 mm, and experience with blood glucose meters suggests that patients find carrying such an object permanently a major inconvenience. Furthermore clinical experience suggests that such devices are very prone to accidental damage in adolescent and young adult patients, and it can be foreseen that the worry of having it lost or stolen, particularly on holiday or away from home, will drive many patients to the considerable expense of purchasing a reserve.

Such a 'permanent companion' has other consequences, and significantly detracts from the initial concept that implantable pumps remove insulin delivery from the need for patient intervention. Thus many patients preferred twice daily to multiple injection therapy not because of the pain or inconvenience of injections, but because they effectively deny their diabetes once having got the injection out of the way (Home et al., 1982). The need to carry the external programmer permanently, its bulky presence in a pocket or handbag, and the need to remember it at every turn, can be expected to prove stressful to some patients. From experience with external infusion pumps this may well be manifest in unexpected ways, such as presumed device dysfunction, damage to the device, or unexplained loss of it.

Cost of Implantable Insulin Infusion Pumps

Assessment of the true costs of producing implantable pumps is not possible at present, for the market is very small and the future uncertain. Thus even the pumps for wider clinical trials are being sold rather than provided to participants, and no doubt the price is set at what the market might be thought to bear, rather than to provide a return on capital. Nevertheless provision of sophisticated mechanical and electronic technology, manufactured to aerospace standards, and packaged in corrosion-free materials, is clearly never going to be cheap, and perhaps never any less expensive than the current UK£8000 for the pump itself.

Discussion of the economics of any disease is complicated, and subject to uncertainties and potential traps. Nevertheless it can be seen that even if the capital and recurrent costs of an implanted pump can be averaged down to UK£3000 a year, the prospects of providing a significant proportion of the 250 000 insulin-treated patients in the UK with such a pump are remote.

Selection of Patients and Circumstances for Application of Implantable Insulin Infusion Pumps

At present the developmental status of implantable pumps is such that the only clear indication for use in patients is for clinical trial purposes, always supposing that this too is ethically justified. It is however reasonable to ask whether any other groups of patients could benefit from their use at the present time, and by what criteria should other patients be selected (or judged suitable to benefit) for their use if the early clinical trials continue to be promising.

Brittle Diabetes

If any group of patients are to be judged as being in need of insulin delivery from implantable devices, then it is first necessary to consider the alternatives. Almost by definition patients who might be considered for this type of pump will already be suffering from very poor control on conventional insulin injection therapy (with maximum educational support), and indeed will generally already be using a multiple injection regimen based on a pen-injector. The decision to consider treatment with a device costing UK£11000 (with accessories), of uncertain safety, and with the considerable surgical, cosmetic, and organisational problems highlighted above, is not taken lightly, but rarely patients have such disastrously controlled diabetes that any potential solution is examined. There is a small group of patients who suffer recurrent admission to hospital, such that all normal social and work activities are destroyed, and with the added risks that come from the emergency management of diabetic ketoacidosis (Gill *et al.*, 1985). This group of patients, often young women from disturbed family backgrounds, are generally believed to be using their diabetes (consciously or otherwise) to relieve other pressures in their lives (Tattersall and Walford, 1985). The use of implanted insulin pumps is then considered as a means of avoiding medical uncertainty over insulin delivery.

Of the other alternatives to insulin injection therapy that have been tried in humans (Table 3), external pumps are open to the same kinds of misuse and disuse in these 'brittle' diabetic patients as are insulin injections. Although pancreas transplantation can be technically successful in some hands, the need for lifetime immunosuppression with its attendant medical risks and need for intensive management make it unsuitable for these patients. Islet transplantation is as yet not technically successful. The use of implanted pumps in brittle diabetes has therefore been attempted for some years, starting with the constant basal rate devices, and at least in some patients gave periods of respite from recurrent hospital admissions (Campbell and Irsigler, 1985).

Nevertheless previous experiences were not without problems, and just because a pump is implanted does not guarantee it cannot be interfered with. At least one pump reservoir was emptied by a patient, while in another interference resulted in pump pocket infections.

Table 3 *Alternative forms of insulin delivery in people with diabetes.*

Insulin injection
        Syringe
        Pen-injectors
External infusion pumps
Implanted infusion pumps
Pancreas transplantation
Islet (cell) transplantation

Clinical Trial Patients

Selection of patients for participation in clinical trials is not without problems, and physicians specializing in diabetes are only too familiar with the pressure from patients to try out new and untried (potentially dangerous) methods of giving insulin, even at considerable expense to themselves. While this partly reflects the inability of physicians to appreciate the behavioural costs of conventional insulin injection therapy, it also is a manifestation of the need of some patients to seek an external solution to their health problems. The impression gained from the use of external pumps is that patients seeking an external solution to their diabetes may be inappropriately attracted to external pumps, with disappointing and sometimes metabolically disasterous results (Bradley *et al.*, 1987).

At present patients chosen for early trials of these new devices are therefore selected largely on the judgment of the study physicians, usually relying on informal personal assessments. Clearly this will not result in a representative group of patients, but often in early studies it is co-operation rather than representativeness that is most needed.

Measuring Outcomes of the Use of Implantable Pumps

If implantable pumps are to be more widely used then, particularly in view of their costs, proof of a useful outcome compared to injection therapy will be important. Classically outcome of diabetes management is measured only in technical terms, mainly relying on blood glucose control often as estimation of glycosylated haemoglobin concentration. Even this however is seriously defective, not only because of the lack of adequate standardization between laboratories and methods, but also because glycosylated haemoglobin only reflects average blood glucose levels through the day, and will not therefore identify the frequency and extent of excursions of blood glucose concentration. Furthermore blood glucose profiles performed at home are subject to timing problems even if laboratory measured, while hospital blood glucose profiles are likely to be unrepresentative of normal eating patterns or activity levels. Blood glucose concentrations are in any case a surrogate for the true outcomes of diabetes, the catastrophic late complications, although the evidence for the relationship between the two has strengthened remarkably in the last five years (Mogensen, 1988).

As far as acute metabolic control is concerned many patients are more interested in hypoglycaemia rates than mean blood glucose level. Again the methods of recording of hypoglycaemia remain unsatisfactory, relying on the patient to remember to record the grade and time of the event on a daily basis. This is a particular problem as many hypoglycaemic episodes may go unrecognized by the patients themselves.

If assessment of metabolic control is not entirely satisfactory for measuring the outcome of new insulin delivery methods, they are at least in advance of measurement of patient well-being. Indeed it is only recently that scales have been developed for assessment of some aspects of quality of life in patients with diabetes (Bradley and Lewis, 1990), while many other aspects remain unaddressed. Furthermore, it has not yet been established whether these instruments have the power to distinguish differences between treatment modalities in fairly small groups of patients.

Conclusions

Implantable insulin infusion pumps remain at an early phase of development, and choice of suitable patients for clinical trial and assessment of outcome remains problematic. Meanwhile, despite the outstanding technical problems and cost, they may be a useful therapeutic option in those rare patients with severely life-disrupting diabetes.

References

Bradley C, Gamsu D S, Moses J L, Knight G, Boulton A J M, Drury J (1987). The use of diabetes specific perceived control and health belief measures to predict treatment choice and efficacy in a feasibility study of continuous subcutaneous insulin infusion pumps. *Psychology and Health* 1: 133–146.

Bradley C, Lewis K S (1990). Measures of psychological well-being and treatment satisfaction developed from the responses of people with tablet-treated diabetes. *Diabetic Medicine* 7: 445–451.

Campbell I W, Irsigler K (1985). Subcutaneous insulin resistance: treatment by implantable device. In, Pickup J C (ed), *Brittle diabetes*. Oxford: Blackwell Scientific. 289–300.

Gill G V, Husband D J, Walford S, Marshall S M, Home P D, Alberti K G M M (1985). Clinical features of brittle diabetes. In, Pickup J C (ed), *Brittle diabetes*. Oxford: Blackwell Scientific. 29–40.

Home P D, Capaldo B, Burrin J M, Worth R, Alberti K G M M (1982). A crossover comparison of continuous subcutaneous insulin infusion (CSII) against multiple insulin injections in insulin-dependent diabetic patients: improved control with CSII. *Diabetes Care* 5: 466–471.

Home P D, Marshall S M (1984). Problems and safety of continuous subcutaneous insulin infusion. *Diabetic Medicine* 1: 41–44.

Irsigler K, Staniszewski K, Regal H (1987). Insulin delivery devices: future outlook. In, Brunetti P, Waldhausl W K (ed), *Advanced models for the therapy of insulin-dependent diabetes*. New York: Raven. 389–393.

Kritz H, Hagmueller G, Lovett R, Irsigler K (1983). Implanted constant basal rate insulin infusion devices for type 1 diabetic patients. *Diabetologia* 23: 78–81.

Mogensen C E (1988). Management of diabetic renal involvement and disease. *Lancet* i: 867–870.

Pickup J C, Keen H, Viberti J C (1980). Continuous subcutnaeous insulin infusion in the treatment of diabetes mellitus. *Diabetes Care* 3: 309–313.

Selam J-L. (1988). Development of implantable insulin pumps: long is the road. *Diabetic Medicine* 5: 724–733.

Slama G, Hautecouverture M, Assan R, Tchobroutsky G (1974). One to seven days continuous intravenous insulin infusion on seven diabetic patients. *Diabetes* 23: 732–738.

Tattersall R B, Walford S. (1985) Brittle diabetes in response to life stress: 'cheating and manipulation'. In, Pickup J C (ed), *Brittle diabetes*. Oxford: Blackwell Scientific. 76–102.

The Pen-Injector's Impact on Self-Management

Judith North

*Head of Voluntary Section, British Diabetic Association, 10
Queen Ann Street. London W1M 0BD, UK.*

Introduction

I write as a former head of the Youth Department at the British Diabetic Association which is responsible for services to youngsters (under the age of 25) with diabetes and their families. I developed a particular interest in teenagers through my involvement in the Youth Diabetes Project (jointly supported by the BDA and Novo-Nordisk) and organising courses for teenagers and their diabetes care professionals. As a head of the BDA Voluntary Section I retain an involvement with the Youth Diabetes Project and Youth Diabetes Groups, plus running training sessions in diabetes for teachers and courses in listening and group skills for clients of all ages with diabetes, and their carers.

On a personal note, I have had Insulin Dependant Diabetes Mellitus (IDDM) since the age of 8, and converted to a multiple injection regimen a few years ago. This has brought a much improved quality of life with valuable flexibility to me (though probably no better 'control'!)

What are Pen-Injectors?

Pen-injection devices for administrating insulin injections are a relatively recent invention. The first device, the Penject appeared about 10 years ago. This consisted of a standard insulin syringe which could be filled with insulin from a bottle and then inserted in a carrier. The carrier included a dial for dialing the required dose. This system was more portable than carrying syringes and bottles but, for adults, would need refilling every couple of days and was a little cumbersome. (However it still remains the only pen system that enables you to know if you have injected or not).

Since 1986, other Pen-injection systems have appeared on the market which contain purpose-made cartridges of insulin which last for several days. These pens heralded the introduction of multiple (that is, more than 2 per day) insulin injection regimens.

Although multiple injection regimens appear to date from the introduction of these pen devices, it should not be forgotten that such regimens for treating insulin dependant diabetes (IDDM) date from the introduction of insulin therapy in 1922. These devices are a product of 20th century technology but multiple doses of insulin are in fact the natural, non-diabetic system of the body producing insulin.

What is the Value of Pen-Injectors?

The advent of Pen-injectors has its impact at the present mainly on young people with diabetes, plus, of course, their parents, schools and the diabetic clinic team. The effects on these groups and their attitudes will influence the self-management of the person with IDDM.

Naturally, many parents are concerned about the future life of their child with diabetes. Since the availability of home blood glucose monitoring (HBGM), parents have been sold the premise that 'good' blood glucose control will prevent the complications of diabetes appearing later in their child's life. Along with this unproven hypothesis, they may also believe that changing to a pen-injection system with multiple doses of insulin will establish 'good control' in their errant teenager.

There are papers to support this (eg McAughey et al, 1986) but there are also an increasing number of workers (eg. Murray et al, 1989) recognising that improving the quality of life can be a more significant gain from a multiple injection system using a pen device.

Impact on Different Groups

Parents

Many parents of youngsters with diabetes feel their child is stigmatized by having to have injections. They may feel being familiar with syringes and needles links them to illegal drugs and the people who use them. From this standpoint, pen-injectors have great advantages – they don't look like syringes and they can't be used to administer other drugs.

The myth that pen-injectors will produce, by magic, 'good control' of diabetes in youngsters, can lead to disappointment when the HbA₁ results are not dramatically different! Often parents who attach stigma and pain to injections may feel a multiple injection regimen with "all those injections" to be dreadful.

Using multiple injections does put the responsibility for diabetes firmly with the person who has the diabetes. Parents may find it difficult to let go of their child's diabetes and to trust that their child's knowledge of diabetes is sound. There can be worries that the flexibility given by a pen-injection system may be abused – for instance, by eating junk food exclusively.

Teachers

Unfortunately, for most teachers, their knowledge of diabetes is scant. On the whole, teachers in training are not even taught first aid and certainly do not get information on how to deal with childhood conditions in the classroom. However, with one child in 500 being affected by diabetes, they are likely to meet at least one child with diabetes in a teaching career.

The myths the general public have about diabetes are also held by the teaching profession. With the advent of the British Diabetic Association (BDA) school pack, as an aid for parents in their role of educating teachers, and diabetes specialist nurses with schools in their remit, the situation is hopefully improving.

Pen-injectors will impact on teachers in several ways. On the plus side, with a pen-injector there will be less need for concern about the timing of sporting activities and meals, and about the content of meals. However, the need for a lunchtime injection brings up problems. For instance, where should the pen be stored? Locking it in the medical room gives problems of access and removes flexibility, but leaving the pen in a pocket or desk could mean the pen could be tried by non-diabetic pupils, or stolen. Obviously education about diabetes can help here, but the dilemmas remain. For anyone without diabetes but with a horror of injections, seeing the process of injecting 'in public' may create additional difficulties.

The Diabetes Care Team

For the diabetes clinic team, the impact of pen-injectors depends on the role of the team member. It will also depend on, of course, the attitude of the individual professional to diabetes and to their clients.

For doctors, on the down side, doctors may feel that they will lose control of their patients in exchange for little improvement in diabetic control. However, the more enlightened clinician may feel that meeting clients with a better quality of life is of great value to the medical profession as well as to the client.

The specialist nurses are likely to be the members of the team who most notice a significantly increased time needed to educate their clients – and also to educate other members of the clinic team. Hopefully this time spent in education will lead to clients having more ability to solve their own problems with diabetes and ultimately relieve this group of professionals from some of the stresses of "not enough hours in the day".

Dietitians may cry out "but they will all eat junk!" The dogmatic members of this profession may miss being able to impose a judgemental system of eating on those with IDDM and miss the simplicity of prescribing set exchanges. There is however, no more reason why someone with diabetes shouldn't eat junk food than someone without diabetes, providing they know what they are doing in terms of estimating when and how much insulin is required. Pen-injectors combined with good education from a client orientated dietitian will facilitate flexible varied eating and minimise the damage of any junk food eaten.

All professionals involved with those having IDDM may fear that they will lose their role for this group of clients and this loss of control may also provoke responses that will need addressing in their professional lives.

The Users

At this moment in time, probably the largest group of people using pen-injectors are the young people with IDDM, young in this case means under 40. Teenagers are a much discussed group and those with diabetes are no exception (North,1990). The impact of pen-injectors on teenagers with diabetes and their effect on self-management though, do illustrate the effects that apply to other groups also.

To be diagnosed as having diabetes when a teenager may be the worst time to be chronically 'ill'. The teenage years herald a period of many changes and though youngsters emerge relatively unscathed, this metamorphosis can be traumatic. To be confronted with a chronic condition at this stage where your body has let you down, and which involves life-style changes does not help to ease any transition.

For youngsters diagnosed as teenagers, and those diagnosed as having insulin dependant diabetes later in life, I find it difficult, personally, to advance reasons to advocate any treatment regimen other than multiple injections with a pen-injector. Perhaps the only possible negative indications are a lack of educational resources or an unwillingness or inability of the person with diabetes to spend time learning about their body's response to insulin and food – and then to put this knowledge into practice. However, from the multiplicity of regimens in use for treating IDDM I must acknowledge different system's suit different people.

A vastly improved quality of life with diabetes can be gained from the flexibility of a pen-injection system and the self-knowledge that taking personal responsibility for self-management brings. Real independence can be gained this way and this is valuable in all aspects of life.

There are some negatives for people *changing* to a pen-injection system however. When life depends on insulin it may be nerve-wracking and stressful to change from drawing up insulin which, in a syringe is very visibly checkable, to relying on a pen to give you the correct dose. It will be necessary to spend more time learning about diabetes and each day will involve more diabetes-related decisions. This can mean diabetes having a higher profile in life, which may be more of a burden.

There have also been instances of doctors prescribing very long acting insulins in large doses that can overlap to give unpredictable and severe hypoglycaemia. This can be worrying, to say the least, to the client. Clients may also be led to believe there is only one long-acting insulin that can be used.

D

Individuals with IDDM do need a certain amount of self-confidence to deal with lunchtime injections and there can be concern about the reactions of other people. It may take time (and contact with someone with diabetes who has 'solved' such problems) to realise that most people don't even notice an injection being given with a pen, and those who do notice are very interested, not negative, horrified or hostile.

Though there has been a focus on using multiple injections for younger clients, it should be realised that the pen device has great value to people who are visually handicapped (see chapter by Porta *et al.* in this book), who have arthritis or who are concerned with the stigma of injections if they need to use injections in later years.

Summary and Conclusions

The pen-injector's impact on self-management of diabetes is to make it firmly SELF-management, which will hopefully be seen as a positive advance in diabetes care both for the client and the medical profession. This can be a help toward seeing diabetes as a deficiency condition requiring manual intervention – not a judgement or retribution from a former life leading to rigid rules for present life.

References

McAughey, E.S, Betts P.J. and Rowe, D.J., (1986) Improved diabetic control on adolescents using the Penject syringe for multiple insulin injections. *Diabetic Medicine* **3**, 234–236

Murray, D.P. *et al.*, (1989) Diabetic Research and Clinical Practice. 7(1):57–60

North, J., (1990) *Teenage Diabetes: What it is and how to get the best out of life* Thorsons & the BDA

3

TECHNOLOGY IN THE PREVENTION AND TREATMENT OF DIABETES COMPLICATIONS

It is in this section that the profound differences in perspectives of different authors is most apparent but we can see the value of multidisciplinary collaboration clearly demonstrated. Great advances have been made in the past decade in the prevention and treatment of a potentially devastating complication, retinopathy. Retinal photography and laser photocoagulation are the most recent technological developments to contribute to progress in this field. Eva Kohner at the Hammersmith Hospital has been at the forefront of these developments. In the first chapter of this section, Richard Newsom, Massimo Porta and Eva Kohner describe the use of these technologies and review the literature evaluating the outcomes associated with the various procedures for retinal screening and treatment. Clearly the focus so far has been firmly on the develoment of the equipment and techniques for screening and treatment. Now, as use of the technology is becoming more widespread, Newsom and his colleagues point out that the focus is broadening to consider the behaviour of the health professionals using the technology, their skills and training and the nature and extent of errors made by different professionals when using the various technologies. It is clear that there is also scope for multidisciplinary studies of patients' responses to different screening programmes, different procedures for recruiting patients, how best to frame information about retinal screening and, indeed, information about complications and screening in general.

Despite the advances made in preventing and treating retinopathy, diabetic retinopathy is still the most common treatable cause of blindness in the UK. The second chapter by Massimo Porta, Alison Bishop and Eva Kohner reviews the many ingenious devices designed to help the visually handicapped to manage their own diabetes. Such devices may offer valuable independence to visually handicapped people with diabetes but may also serve to reduce valued social support if a reduction in the number of visits from community nurses is one consequence of that independence. As the authors point out, the pros and cons of the new devices and the implications of their use have yet to be fully explored.

Chris Stiles provides a thought provoking third chapter in this section. New developments such as total contact casting and new surgical techniques which have facilitated progress in treating diabetic foot ulcers and other complications of the feet are described. As was the case with developments in retinal screening described by Newsom and colleagues, one of the main issues for chiropody is how best to use professional skills, and concerns about inappropriately trained personnel undertaking procedures that may be dangerous in unskilled hands. There is cause for concern that the relatively low tech profession of chiropody is insufficiently valued in high tech medicine. When chiropodists are not properly included as full members of the diabetes care team, the real potential of chiropodists will not be realised. Stiles argues that not only does the chiropodist have special skills for managing problems of the feet but is also able to play an important role in educating people with diabetes and to offer that valuable and all too rare commodity, a listening ear.

The final chapter in this section is by John Kramer, Alan Jacobson, Chris Ryan, William Murphy and other members of the group involved with the Diabetes Control and Complications Trial. The DCCT is currently being undertaken to establish the extent to which maintenance of near-normal blood glucose control will reduce the onset or progression of microvascular complications of diabetes. The psychological effects of the treatment regimens are being studied and the measures employed are described. The need to encourage patients to keep up the very considerable effort needed to maintain tight control of blood glucose levels has meant that the DCCT has had to tackle the difficult questions of how best to select, recruit and motivate the patients in the study. Although different selection, recruitment and motivation procedures were not the focus of study and have not been evaluated in a controlled manner, they have been carefully considered and developed and explicitly described in a manner that is unique in diabetes research. The experience gained in running the DCCT offers valuable insights for other researchers planning clinical trials, and health professionals concerned with how to motivate the patients in their clinics.

Use and Evaluation of Technology in the Detection and Treatment of Diabetic Retinopathy

Richard B. S. Newsom, Massimo Porta and Eva. M. Kohner

Diabetic Retinopathy Unit, Dept. Medicine, Royal Postgraduate Medical School, Du Cane Road, London W12 0NN, UK.

Introduction

Diabetic retinopathy is the major cause of visual loss in people with diabetes. At present no medical treatment can prevent its development or progression. Only photocoagulation has been found to be effective in arresting and reversing the development of sight threatening lesions. These lesions often develop in the absence of visual symptoms, so our main aim is to detect the and treat retinopathy before it becomes sight threatening. The difference between detection and retinal assessment should be born in mind when approaching this subject. The most accurate and sensitive methods for diagnosing retinopathy will not necessarily be suitable when screening, as they are costly and time consuming.

Screening

There are an estimated 2,000,000 people with diabetes in the U.K. (Kohner 1978). Of these 17.4/1000 per year are likely to develop background retinopathy and 5.8/1000 per year will progress to sight threatening retinopathy (Dwyer et al., 1985; Rohan et al., 1989). Diabetic retinopathy is the most common cause of blindness between the ages of 19–65 in the UK (Sorsby, 1972). In the USA about 5000 cases of blindness related to diabetes are reported annually (National Institute of Health Publication, 1980). Many of these people are relatively young when they go blind, so the social and economic cost is high. The regular screening of diabetic patients is essential, as early retinopathy is symptomless and may progress rapidly. The aim of screening is twofold; 1. to diagnose sight threatening retinopathy which will need urgent referral for treatment; 2. to diagnose mild retinopathy, which does not need referral, but does need regular follow up in the screening clinic. The cost effectiveness of screening and treatment programmes have been clearly shown (Foulds *et al.*, 1983; Bron 1985; Javitt *et al.*, 1989), however there are few really effective programmes in place and preventable disasters still regularly occur. The debate is not only about which technologies are the most effective but about who should be using them.

1. Direct Ophthalmoscopy

Although the ophthalmoscope is the most common tool used to assess the retina it is clear that retinoscopy is a specialist skill. Palmberg and Smith (1981) compared direct ophthalmoscopy performed by board certified ophthalmologists with retinal photography and fluroscein angiography in the detection of early retinopathy. He found that ophthalmoscopy was on average 10% less sensitive than photography, though this difference was smaller in severe retinopathy.

The story is very different if the observers have not received specific training. Sussman *et al.* (1982) showed that doctors with no such training were very poor at detecting retinopathy. Under ideal conditions junior doctors made serious errors in the diagnosis of retinopathy in 70% of cases. Training improves recognition, so that senior medical internists made serious errors in 52% and diabetologists in 50% of cases. This compared with 9% by general ophthalmologists and 0% by retinal experts, who were able to use both direct and indirect ophthalmoscopy.

A similar UK study showed that a Consultant Physician missed 49% of cases with background retinopathy and 28% of cases with proliferative retinopathy, when compared with retinal photography. A nurse specialist missed retinopathy in 50% of cases with background retinopathy (Forrest *et al.*, 1987). These figures are very high and may, in part, be explained by the overgrading of retinal photographs by the graders, a common problem in all comparison studies. Clinically significant retinopathy may not be missed quite so frequently. However these studies stress the need to train fully prospective ophthalmoscopists.

Foulds *et al.* (1985) suggested that there is no difference between the accuracy of referral from trained physicians or ophthalmologists for severe diabetic retinopathy but this study was weakened by not using retinal photography as an objective assessment of retinopathy.

The importance of pupillary dilation, when examining eyes for retinopathy, cannot be over emphasised. Klein *et al.* (1985) showed that ophthalmoscopy through undilated pupils is a particularly insensitive and nonspecific method of detecting and classifying retinopathy. Retinal experts failed to detect proliferative retinopathy in 45% of cases and misgraded background retinopathy in 54% of cases.

Much has been made of the role of opticians in the screening of diabetic patients, as they are trained to recognise retinopathy and are of easier access to patients than hospital clinics. Burns-Cox and Dean Heart (1985) assessed an opticians based screening service and argued that it was a reasonable alternative to hospital clinics. In their study, opticians only missed 5% of patients with diabetic retinopathy through undilated pupils. This study is flawed by the use of clinic ophthalmologists and not retinal photography as a method of detecting retinopathy, so a comparative detection rate cannot be derived.

Although the direct ophthalmoscope is a relatively insensitive tool for the diagnosis of retinopathy it does have the advantage of being widely available, portable and inexpensive. It gives good magnification and the inclusion of a green filter in many models means that the retinal vessels and new vessels are more clearly seen. However it does suffer from some disadvantages: it gives a small field of view (8°), (Lee, 1990), a poor view of the periphery of the retina, it does not give a stereoscopic view of the retina (and therefore is of little use in assessing macular oedma), and of producing no objective permanent record. Extensive training is required before the operator can be confident in using the direct ophthalmoscope as a screening tool, a fact that most medical schools do not appreciate.

The conclusion from these studies is that direct ophthalmoscopy can therefore be used as a screening method under certain circumstances: 1. That the examiners are fully trained; 2. That the pupils are fully dilated; 3. If only a gross classification of retinopathy is required; 4. That retinopathy detected by this method is referred for specialist evaluation.

2. Retinal Photography

A. Non-mydriatic photography

An important development has been the non-mydriatic camera, already in use for mass screening in general diabetic clinics or community projects (figure 1).

Klein *et al.* (1985) compared the non-mydriatic camera with the normal fundus camera. Using Kodachrome film in both, exact agreement between the two cameras was found on 82.5% of occurances. This increased to 86% when the pupils were dilated. However there was a greater likelihood of undercalling the grade of retinopathy, and more of the photographs were ungradeable using the non-mydriatic camera (12.7% compared with the standard camera 2.0%). This compares well with the other methods of screening discussed above, and the authors concluded that the non-mydriatic camera may be of value in the routine screening of diabetic patients in areas where ophthalmologic care or physician availability is limited.

A similar conclusion was reached by Mohan *et al.* (1988) in their evaluation of the non-mydriatic camera in Indian and European patients. They found the Canon CR3 was a reasonable screening tool in both populations although it had some significant drawbacks. Six percent of the photographs were unassessable and another 12% were only of limited use. Difficulties were found in the elderly patients, due to small pupillary diameters, and those who

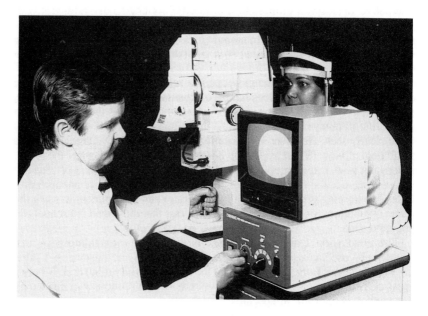

Figure 1. The Non-mydriatic Camera.

had cataracts, though iris colour had no significant effect on the quality of the photographs. Early referral of the patients with unassessable photographs was recommended to check for retinopathy and other concurrent ocular disease. The camera was also of limited use in the detection and assessment of maculopathy, because the retinal 'thickness' could not be evaluated. Therefore the importance of the testing of visual acuity, for the detection of clinically significant maculopathy, was emphasised. The camera used a very bright flash and caused significant discomfort to the patients.

The non-mydriatic camera fails to detect lesions outside the 45° field, this occured in 4% of cases seen by Mohan *et al.* (1988), though in other studies higher figures of 8–15% of cases have been recorded. Klein *et al.* (1985) suggested that 27% of proliferative diabetic retinopathy occurs outside the area normally covered by the non-mydriatic camera an observation supported by Barrie and MacCuish (1986). This is clearly a major disadvantage as haemorrhage from such new vessels can lead to blindness.

Ryder *et al.* (1985) compared the Canon CR2-45N and the CR3-45N, (the main difference being the minimum pupillary size needed to take gradeable photographs) with direct ophthalmoscopy by clinic physicans. The CR3 produced fair to good pictures 73% of the time, compared with 37% for the CR2. The detection rate of retinopathy was 4x higher than ophthalmoscopy through undilated pupils and 2x higher than through dilated pupils. Again this study failed to compare the non-mydriatic camera with the standard camera. They therefore diagnosed retinopathy in fewer of their clinic patients than other similar studies, and made no comment on the training given to their clinic ophthalmoscopists. Williams *et al.* (1986) compared the Kowa or Canon CR3 with a clinic doctor and a ophthalmologist. They found the non-mydriatic camera gave a false negative of 6.8% and a false positive rate of 2%.

Another source of criticism for the non-mydriatic camera is that Polaroid film is often used. This film has a poor resolution and may not be able to detect early new vessel changes. Jones *et al.* (1988) reported that up to 20% of their Polaroid prints could not be assessed due to poor quality. This compared with 2.4% with the standard camera. A recent German report (Chantelau *et al.*, 1989) suggests that a single 45° fundus Polaroid print per patient may suffice for screening purposes. However the report recommended that if any retinopathy is detected the patient should be immediately referred to an ophthalmologist for expert advice.

The non-mydriatic camera is not without its drawbacks. It is expensive, in normal use it gives only one field of view and poor magnification. Intercurrent eye disease, such as cataracts, leads to a high failure rate. The lack of stereopsis makes the assessment of macular oedema impossible. The camera is of most use in district screening programmes, for elderly diabetic patients who find clinic attendance difficult. Elderly patients are more likely to have cateracts or macular oedema thus limiting the usefulness of this camera for screening this group.

The benefits are: that patients can be screened with undilated pupils; that the camera is easy to use; it is sensitive and specific for retinopathy; it produces a large field of view which compares well with the standard camera; it gives a permanent record of the retina; it is transportable and relatively cheap to run.

B. Mydriatic photography

Seven field, 30°, colour, stereoscopic, retinal photography through pharmacologically dilated pupils, is the gold standard by which other technologies are compared. Photographs are taken using a standard retinal camera and fine grain colour transparency film. The photographs are graded using the modified Airlie house (The Diabetic Retinopathy Study Research Group, 1981) system of photographic grading. The number of microaneurysms, and haemorrhages on each photograph are counted and they are also compared to several standard photographs to grade exudate, cotton wool spots, new vessels, retinitis proliferans and photocoagulation scars. This technique although sensitive is rarely used for screening as it may take 20 minutes to grade even the photographs from 1 eye, and so is too slow for general clinic work. More recently it has been shown that analysis of only 4 fields gives a sensitivity of 90% (Moss *et al.*, 1989).

Fluorescein angiography is arguably the most sensitive test for retinopathy. A recent study showed that 21% of patients, without retinopathy as diagnosed on photography, had evidence of microaneurysms with fluorescein angiography (The Diabetes Control and Complications Trial, 1987). However 19% of those with no retinopathy with fluorescein had some evidence with photography. They concluded that fluorescein angiography when used in conjunction with colour photography, allowed a modest increase in sensitivity to the earliest signs of diabetic retinopathy, which are clinically unimportant but useful in a research context. Palmberg and Smith (1981) showed little difference between the two techniques arguing that many lesions diagnosed as microaneurysms on the fluorescein angiogram were artifacts, matching with retinal pigment epithelial defects, when colour photographs were reviewed. This argument will not apply in a clinical setting because the lesions appear at a characteristic time in the photographic sequence.

The advantages of the standard camera is that it produces good quality, stereoscopic retinal photographs with a reasonable magnification. These can be accurately assessed using internationally standardised grading techniques. New vessels and macular oedema are easily visualised because of stereoscopic pictures produced and a permanent record of the retinopathy status can be kept in the patient's notes. The results from the photography may also be discussed with the patient and can make a significant contribution to the patient's education about their disease. These features make the standard retinal camera an excellent research tool. Fluorescein angiography and retinal photography are essential for retinal assessment in clinical practice, and some European countries recommend them as methods of screening. However they are costly, time consuming procedures demanding highly skilled staff and good hospital based backup facilities, and so are generally reserved for research in specialist establishments.

3. Other Methods of Retinal Examination

A. *Indirect ophthalmoscopy*

Indirect ophthalmoscopy with a 20 dioptre (D) lens yields a clear view of most of the retina and is less troubled by lens and vitreous opacities than the direct ophthalmoscope. Studies using both the direct and indirect ophthalmoscope show a large improvement in detection rate. Moss *et al.* (1985) showed that in the case of retinal experts there was an 86% agreement with retinal photography. They missed 26% of patients with proliferative retinopathy, but argued that only one eye with 'high risk' characteristics was missed. In an interesting report Ferris and Sackett (1983) showed how effective this technique could be. A nurse practitioner was trained in the visualisation of the fundi and the grading of diabetic retinopathy. In a prospective study of 90 patients, no patient with serious retinopathy was missed, although minor grading errors were made in 22% of cases.

The advantages of the 20D are: that a clear view of the retina is obtained, the field of view is large (57.1°), and that anatomical relations are preserved. The disadvantages are: that the technique is difficult to use and that it gives little magnificaton (x3) (early lesions, new vessels and intra retinal microangiopathy are therefore easily overlooked). Furthermore it yields no permanent record. The 20D lens is a good tool for the screening of retinopathy, and if the experience of Ferris and Sackett could be reproduced, highly accurate screening for diabetic patients would be available without referal to ophthalmologists.

B. Slit lamp based

Slit lamp biomicroscopy with magnification using specialist lenses gives the clinician a good three-dimensional view of the retina; vital for the assessment of the macula and macular lesions. The 90D has been popular for some years giving a good magnification (x7.7) of the retina in return for a rather small field of view (37°). The newer 78D and 60D lenses have bigger magnification (x9.6), but a smaller field of view (29°), and so are becoming popular. The latest 150D lens gives an excellent field of view (60°) and a reasonable magnification (x5.2). With this lens the whole retina may be visualised, and so this will be a very powerful tool for retinal examination (Blaire Lee, 1990). These lenses may eventually replace the 20D lens for retinal assessment as they give better magnification and yet maintain a good field of view.

In a recent Swedish study the sensitivity of indirect ophthalmoscopy using 60D, enhanced slit lamp examination was compared to using non stereoscopic photography of the posterior pole. Screening for retinitis proliferans and for maculopathy was undertaken. In both series the photography proved superior to the slit lamp examination in sensitivity and speed (Kalm et al., 1989 and 1989a).

The drawbacks of this type of screening are many, the technique is time consuming, costly, dependant on skilled personnel, and so may be more suited to retinal assessment in a specialist clinic. Other methods such as colour discrimination, contrast sensitivity, electrodiagnostic tests, and vitreous fluorophotometry have all been used as methods to assess retinal function. However they are time consuming, costly and do not relate to the anatomical progression of the disease. They are therefore not suitable for screening purposes.

Conclusion

For a disease to be suitable for screening, several criteria need to be met:

1. The disease should appear within a defined population and represent a significant health problem;
2. Screening techniques should be: sensitive, specific, cheap, widely available, easy to administer, cost effective and cause little psychological or physical discomfort to the patient.
3. There should be an effective treatment for the disease.

All these criteria are met in diabetic retinopathy. Screening programmes are essential if retinopathy is to be effectively treated. The cheapest and most widely available technique is direct ophthalmoscopy, but it should be used through dilated pupils and with a well trained operator. The non-mydriatic camera is a reasonable alternative providing a sensitive permanent record of the patient's retina. Another promising avenue is the training of clinical assistants and paramedical staff in indirect ophthalmoscopy and slit lamp biomicroscopy to screen large numbers of patients with the high accuracy that these techniques afford.

Treatment of Retinopathy

Laser photocoagulation is the only effective method of treating sight threatening retinopathy, but unfortunately it does not guarantee maintenance of good vision. The technologies for retinal photocoagulation were developed during the 1960s. Early reports showed this technique to be effective on local lesions and using scattered photocoagulation new vessels at the disc could be resolved (Dobree and Taylor, 1968). There is still debate as to which method of treatment is the most effective, what type of treatment should be given, when and how much. There is also some evidence that tight metabolic control can slow the progression of the disease (Doft *et al.*, 1984; Klein *et al.*, 1984; Lauritizen *et al.*, 1982; KROC 1984), and that certain drugs may have a small effect. However, in themselves, these cannot be regarded as treatments and as such lie outside the scope of this chapter (DAMAD 1989; Frank *et al.*, 1984).

Technologies of photocoagulation

Xenon arc

The Xenon arc was first developed by Meyer-Schwickerath (1959). He developed a system to focus sunlight directly on to the retina of his patients. This was later replaced by an electrical 'white light' source. It was found to be effective in the treatment of retinopathy, reversing the signs of retinal ischaemia such as venous beading, cotton wool spots, and new vessels

(Dobree and Taylor, 1968; British Multicenter Group, 1977). Light from the Xenon arc is delivered through a direct ophthalmoscope. This requires a retrobulbar anaesthetic to immobilise the eye, causes large visual field defects by destroying the full thickness of the retina and causes discomfort to the patient. Because of these drawbacks most units now base their treatment around the argon laser. However the xenon arc is still of use if new vessels persist in spite of argon laser treatment.

Laser Photocoagulation

Argon laser

In 1969 L'Esperance developed the argon blue/green laser. The wavelengths of light from this laser are well absorbed by haemoglobin (488 & 514 nm) and so are more efficient and cause less discomfort to the patient. The argon laser delivers a wide range of laser power (0–100m watts) and spot sizes (100–1000µm), giving the Laser a great flexibility in treatment.

A major problem with the original argon laser is the strength of the aiming beam. Heavy users found that their macula pigment was affected by the intense laser light. This was rectified by removing the blue light from the aiming beam. The green argon laser is also used to treat patients' macula, because of fears that the intense blue light may cause excessive damage, as it is absorbed by the patient's foveal pigment (Cruess et al., 1988).

Krypton laser

The krypton laser (647nm) causes minimal damage to the inner retinal layers. It is not absorbed by xanthophyll or oxyhaemoglobin, but by the melanin in the retinal pigment epithelium. It is useful in the treatment of subretinal vessels, and subretinal neovascular membranes, although it has also been employed for panretinal photocoagulation.

Dye laser

The variable-wavelength dye laser, capable of reaching a specific level in the retina or choroid, has offered exciting new developments, and it promises soon to be part of the ophthalmologist's armament in the treatment of eye disease (Bessette and Nguyen 1989).

Diode laser

This interesting new development uses the infra-red band of light. The laser is small compared with the argon or the dye. It is easily transportable and slots on to a normal slit lamp. The diode laser produces a relatively slow blanching of the retina, compared with the argon laser. It is considerably cheaper than the argon laser and does not need to be air or water cooled like its predecessors.

However it is more uncomfortable for the patients. There are not as yet clinical studies comparing the efficacy of the diode with the argon laser, however as it works on the same principle as other lasers, the efficacy will probably be similar (McHugh *et al.*, 1989).

Methods of Treatment

Panretinal photocoagulation

The technique of panretinal photocoagulation (PRP), was developed in the 1970s. It is used for the treatment of new vessels, the aim being to reduce the amount of ischaemic retina so reducing the drive to produce new vessels. It was shown to be an effective treatment by the Diabetic Retinopathy Study (DRS) (1978).

The laser may be delivered via a slit lamp using a Goldman three mirror, a Rodenstock panfundoscope, or a 90 or a 78 D lens. The advantage of a three mirror lens is that the far periphery of the retina can be treated but the localisation of the macula is difficult and may lead to macular burns. The Rodenstock lens gives a clear view of the whole fundus and is therefore safer to use than the three mirror and PRP may be delivered faster. Laser therapy may also be delivered by an indirect ophthalmoscope using a 20 D lens, giving the operator more flexibility but less control. Between 1500–4000 burns are given covering the retina but sparing the macula (fig. 2). During PRP the recommended size is 500μm as larger sizes cause anterior chamber damage. The laser burns are placed 1–1.5 burn diameters away from each other, and the meridian in both the nasal fields should be avoided as this preserves the visual field. This is now of great importance in view of the Driving Vehicle Licensing Centre's new visual field regulations. Although the maximum number of burns is usually about 4000 it has been shown that up to 11,513 burns can be given without losing central vision (Aylward *et al.*, 1989). Panretinal photocoagulation has some occasional side effects which include: reactive macular oedema leading to a 1 or 2 line reduction in visual acuity (Meyers, 1980), corneal erosion, lens denaturation, choriovitreal proliferations, subretinal neovascular membranes and a reduction in visual field.

The first study to show conclusively the effectiveness of PRP was the Diabetic Retinopathy Study (DRS). This study assessed the efficacy of the argon laser and the Xenon Arc for the treatment of proliferative retinopathy (DRS, 1978). The trial showed, that after 4 months of follow up of eyes with proliferative retinopathy, eyes treated with panretinal photocoagulation had a 8% chance of suffering severe visual loss, while in the untreated eye this was 30%. The study also found that eyes treated with argon laser faired slightly better than those treated with Xenon arc. This result was challenged by Okun (1981) who suggested that this discrepancy was due to faulty technique. In his study of 2688 patients he found a severe complication rate of only 13%, at 72 months, less than the DRS figure for argon laser. He also commented that the increased complication rate in the xenon group could have been due to a larger

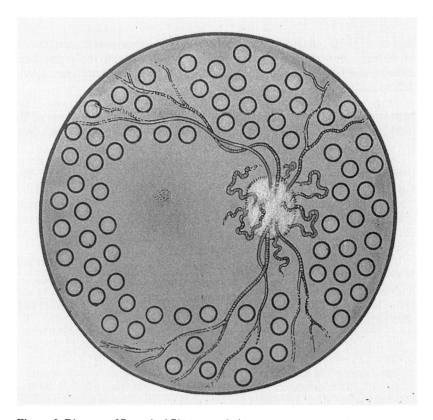

Figure 2. Diagram of Panretinal Photocoagulation.

amount of treatment given in this group rather than a difference between the treatments themselves. The British Multicenter Study (1984) confirmed the benefit of Xenon arc treatment. There is evidence that the benefits of photocoagulation treatment are sustained for several years. Little (1985) found that 67% of eyes had vision of 20/50 or better at 10–12 years after argon laser treatment. Sullivan *et al.* (in press) found that 83% of patients maintained good vision in their better eye after 10 years of follow up.

Schulenburg *et al.* (1979) compared the argon and the krypton lasers for PRP and found comparable results but the krypton laser produced smaller field defects. Blankenship *et al.* (1989) found that krypton PRP preserved visual acuity in 84% of patients compared with 79% treated with argon laser. In view of it's absorption pattern Krypton laser has been used to treat subretinal neovascular membranes close to the fovea with some success (Decker *et al.*, 1984).

Macular treatment

Patz *et al.* (1973) identified macular oedma as 'the overlooked complication in diabetic retinopathy'. They pioneered treatment with the argon laser showing that both treatment of local lesions and grid treatment (figure 3) of a diffuse maculopathy produced excellent results.

To give an effective macular grid 50–200 burns are given, the size of the burn is reduced to 100 μm, to decrease the field loss, and the duration of the burn is shortened to 0.06s to reduce retinal damage. Local treatment is effective when leaking vessels or microaneurysms are causing maculopathy.

Patz *et al.* (1973) reported that 95% of their treated patients maintained or improved their vision, as compared to only 36% of the control group. The Early Treatment Diabetic Retinopathy Study (1985) has recently reported that 'focal photocoagulation of clinically significant macular oedema substantially reduces the risk of visual loss'. They showed that 50% of the treated patients did better than the control group after 12 months and, at all stages of the disease treatment, made a significant improvement to the visual outcome.

The Xenon arc has also been used to treat macular oedma. The British Multicenter Study Group (1983) found that treated eyes saw on average 2.7 lines better than the untreated eyes after 7 years. Generally focal treatment was given but no specific protocol for treatment was made. Davies *et al.* (1989) showed that these beneficial effects were maintained for 10 years.

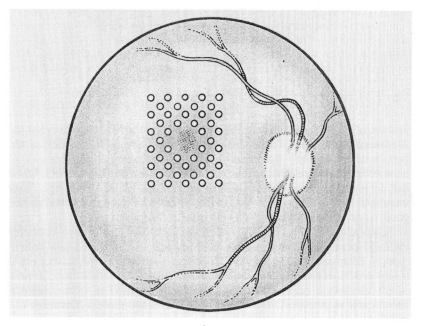

Figure 3. Diagram of local treatment.

Summary and Conclusions

Effective treatment for diabetic retinopathy is still based on the destruction of ischaemic peripheral retina which reduces the visual field and potentially causes a variety of sight damaging complications. The development of effective treatment for the earlier stages of the disease must be the prime objective for future research. Until that time a serious commitment to screening using well trained, highly motivated staff should be made. The provision of such staff and equipment is essentially a political decision. However they should be readily accessable to diabetic patients in all districts, and should be able to refer patients to well organised eye clinics for rapid assessment and treatment. The failure of such a provision in many parts of the country is the reason that diabetic retinopathy still remains the most common treatable cause of blindness.

References

Aiello, L.M., Beethan, W.P., Baodimos, M.S., Chazan, B.I. and Bradley, B.F. (1969). Ruby laser photocoagulation in the treatment of proliferative diabetic retinopathy. In N. Goldman and S. Fine, *Treatment of diabetic retinopathy.* 437–463 United States Department of Health

Aylward, G.W., Pearson, R.V., Jagger, J.D. and Hamilton, A.M. (1989). Extensive argon laser photocoagulation in the treatment of proliferative diabetic retinopathy. *British Journal of Ophthalmology* 73, 2013–2015

Barrie, T. and MacCuish, A.C. (1986). letter *British Medical Journal* 293, 1304–1305

Bessette, F.M. and Nguyen, L. (1989). Laser light: its nature and its action on the eye. *Canadian Medical Association Journal* 141, 1141–8

Blankenship, G.W., Gerke, E. and Battle, J.F. (1989). Red krypton and blue-green argon laser diabetic panretinal photocoagulation. *Graefes Archives of Clinical and Experimental Ophthalmology* 227, 364–368

British Multicenter Study Group. (1984). Photocoagulation for proliferative retino-pathy: A randomised controlled study using the Xenon-arc. *Diabetalogia* 26, 109–115

British Multicenter Study Group. (1983). Photocoagulation for diabetic maculopathy: a randomised controlled clinical trial using the Xenon Arc. *Diabetes* 32, 1010–1016

Bron, A.J. (1985). Screening for treatable retinopathy. *British Medical Journal* 290, 1025–1026

Burns-Cox, C.J. and Dean Hart, J.C. (1985). Screening of diabetics for retinopathy by ophthalmic opticians. *British Medical Journal* 290, 1052–1054

Chantelau, E., Zwecker, M., Weiss, H., Kluxen, G. and Berger, M. (1989). Fundus Polaroid screening for diabetic retinopathy. Is one print per patient enough? *Diabetes Care* 12, 223–226

Cruess, A.F., Williams, J.C. and Willan, A.R. (1988). Argon green and krypton red laser treatment of diabetic macular edema. *Canadian Journal of Ophthalmology* 23, 262–266

DAMAD Study Group. (1989). Effect of Aspirin alone and Aspirin and Dipyridamole in Early diabetic retinopathy. A preliminary multicenter trial. *Diabetes* 38, 491–498

Davies, E.G., Petty, R.G. and Kohner, E.M. (1989). Long term effectiveness of photocoagulation for diabetic maculopathy. *Eye* 3, 764–767

Decker, W.L., Grabowski, W.M. and Annesley, W.H. Jr. (1984). Krypton red laser photocoagulation of subretinal neovascular membranes located within the Foveal Avascular Zone. *Ophthalmology* 91, 1582–1586

Diabetes Control and Complications Trial Group. (1987). Color photography versus fluorscein angiography in the diabetes control trial. *Archives of Ophthalmology* 105, 1344–1351

Diabetic Retinopathy Study and Research Group. (1978). Photocoagulation treatment of proliferative diabetic retinopathy: The second report of study findings. *Ophthalmology* 85, 82–106

Diabetic Retinopathy Study and Research Group:. (1981). A modification of the Airlie House classification of diabetic retinopathy. Diabetic Retinopathy Study Report No. 7. *Investigative Ophthalmology and Visual Sciences* 21, 210

Dobree, J.H. and Taylor, E. (1968). Treatment of proliferative diabetic retinopathy by repeated light coagulation. *Transactions of the Ophthalmology Society* U.K. 8, 313–329

Doft, B.H., Kingsley, L.A. and Orchard, T.F. (1984). The association between long term diabetic control and early retinopathy. *Ophthalmology* 91, 763–769

Dwyer, M.S., Melton, J.L. III, Ballard, D.J., Pasquale, J., Palumbo, L.J., Trautman, J.C. *et al.* (1985). Incidence of diabetic retinopathy and blindness: A population-based study in Rochester Minnesota. *Diabetes Care* 8, 316–322

Early Treatment Diabetic Retinopathy Study (1985). Report No.1 Photocoagulation for diabetic macular edema. *Archives of Ophthalmology* 103, 1796–1806

Ferris, F. and Sackett, L., (1983). Management of retinal vascular and macula disorders. In S.L. Fine & S.L. Owens, *Screening for diabetic retinopathy*. Williams & Wilkins, London

Forrest, R.D., Jackson, C.A. and Yudkin, J.S. (1987). Screening for diabetic retinopathy- Comparison of a nurse and doctor with retinal photography. *Diabetes Research* 5, 39–42

Foulds, S.W., McCuish, A. and Barrie, T. (1985). The cost effectiveness of screening for diabetic eye disease. *Seminars in Ophthalmology* 2, 45–50

Foulds, W.S., McCuish, A., Barrie, T., Green, F., Scobie, I.N., Ghafourr, I.M., *et al.* (1983). Diabetic retinopathy in the West of Scotland. Its detection and prevalence, and the cost effectiveness of a proposed screening program. *Health Bulletin* 6, 318–326

Frank, R.N., Keirn, R.J. and Schofield, P.J. (1984). Galactose induced retinal capillary basement membrane thickening. Prevented by Sorbinil. *Investigative Ophthalmology and Visual Sciences* 24, 1519–1524

Javitt, J.C., Canner, J.K. and Sommer, A. (1989). Cost effectiveness of current approaches to the control of retinopathy in type 1 diabetes. *Ophthalmology.* 95, 225–264

Jones, D., Dolben, J., Owens, D.R., Owens, D.R., Vora, J.P., Young, S. *et al.* (1988). Non-mydriatic Polaroid photography in screening for diabetic retinopathy: Evaluation in a clinical setting. *British Medical Journal* 296, 1029–1030

Kalm, H., Egertsen, R. and Blohme, G. (1989). Non-stereo fundus photography as a screening procedure for diabetic retinopathy among patients with type II diabetes. Compared with 60D enhanced slit-lamp examination. *Acta Ophthalmologica Copenhagen* 67, 546–553

Kalm, H., Sjodell, L. and Jonsson, R. (1989). Non-stereo photographic screening after panretinal photocoagulation for proliferative diabetic retinopathy. Compared with 60D enhanced slit-lamp examination. *Acta Ophthalmologica Copenhagen* **67**, 554–559

Klein, R., Klein, B.E.K., Neider, M.W., Hubbard, L.D., Meuer, S.M., and Brothers, R.J. (1985). Diabetic retinopathy as detected using ophthalmoscopy, a nonmydriatic camera and a standard fundus camera. *Ophthalmology* **92**, 485–491

Kohner, E.M. *(1978)*. *Transactions of the Ophthalmology Society* **98**, 299

KROC Collaborative Study Group. (1984). Blood glucose control and the evolution of diabetic retinopathy and albuminuria. A preliminary multicenter trial. *New England Journal of Medicine* **311**, 365–372

L'Esperance, F.A. (1969). The treatment of ophthalmic vascular disease by argon laser photocoagulation. *Transactions of the American Academy of Ophthalmology and Otolaryngology* **73**, 1077–1096

Lauritizen, T., Deckert, T. and Sterno Study group. (1983). Effect of one years near normal blood glucose levels on retinopathy in insulin dependent diabetes melitus. *Lancet* **(i)** 200–204

Lee, N. B. (1990). Biomicroscopic examination of the ocular fundus with a +150 dioptre lens. *British Journal of Ophthalmology* **74**, 294–296

Little, H.L.. (1985). Long term results of argon laser photocoagulation. *Ophthalmology* **92**, 279–283

McHugh, J.D., Marshall, J., Ffytche, T.J., Hamilton, A.M., Raven, A. and Keeler, C.R. (1989) Initial clinical experience using a Diode Laser in the treatment of retinal vascular disease. *Eye* **3**, 516–517

Meyer-Schwickerath, G. (1959). *Lichtcoagulation*. Stuttgart, Enke Verlag

Meyers, S.M. (1980). Macular edema after scatter laser photocoagulation for proliferative diabetic retinopathy. *American Journal of Ophthalmology* **90**, 210–216

Mohan, R., Kohner, E.M., Aldington, S.J., Nijhar, I., Mohan, V. and Mather, J.M. (1988). Evaluation of a non-mydriatic camera in Indian and European diabetic patients. *British Journal of Ophthalmology* **72**, 294–296

Moss, S.E., Klein, R. and Kessler, S.D. (1985). Comparison between ophthalmoscopy and fundus photography in determining the severity of diabetic retinopathy. *Ophthalmology* **92**, 62–67

Moss, S.E., Meuer, S.M., Klein, R., Hubbard, L.D., Brothers, R.J. and Klein, B.E.K (1989). Are seven standard photographic fields necessary for classification of diabetic retinopathy? *Investigative Ophthalmology and Visual Sciences* **30**, 823–828

National Institutes of Health publication (1980). *Diabetes, a national plan to reduce the mortality and morbidity.* **81**, 2284

Okun, E., Johnson, G.P., Boniuk, I., Arribas, N.P., Escoffery, R.F. and Grand, M.G. (1981) A review of 2688 consective eyes in the format of the Diabetic Retinopathy study. *Ophthalmology.* **91**, 1458–1463

Palmberg, P. and Smith, M. (1981). The natural history of retinopathy in insulin dependent juvenile-onset diabetics. *Ophthalmology* **88**, 613–618

Patz, A., Schatz, H. and Berkow, J.W. (1973) Macula edema an overlooked complication of diabetic retinopathy. *Transactions of the American Academy of Ophthalmology and Otolaryngology* **77**, 34–42

Rohan, T.E., Frost, C.D. and Wald, N.T. (1989). Prevention of blindness by screening for diabetic retinopathy; a quantative assessment. *British Medical Journal* **299**, 1198–1201

Ryder, R.E.J., Young, S., Vora, J.P., Atiea, J.A., Owens, J.R. and Hayes J.M. (1985).

Screening for diabetic retinopathy using poloroid retinal photography through undilated pupils. *Practical Diabetes* **2**, 34–39

Schulenburg, W.E., Hamilton, A.M. and Blach, R.K. (1979). A comparitive study of argon laser and krypton laser in the treatment of diabetic disc neovascularisation. *British Journal of Ophthalmology* **63**, 412–417

Sorsby, A. (1972). The incidence and causes of blindness in England and Wales 1963–68. DHSS report on Public health and medical subjects. No. 128 London HMSO. 44

Sullivan, P., Caldwell, G., Alexander, N. and Kohner, E.M. (1990). Long term outcome after photocoagulation for proliferative diabetic retinopathy. *Journal of the American Medical Association* : in press

Sussman, E.J., Tsiaras, W.G. and Soper, K.A.. (1982). Diagnosis of diabetic eye disease. *Journal of the American Medical Association* **247**, 3231–3234

Williams, R., Nussey, S., Humphry, R. and Thompson, G. (1986). Assessment of non-mydriatic fundus photography in detection of diabetic retinopathy. *British Medical Journal* **293**, 1304–1305

Aids to Diabetes Management for the Visually Handicapped

Massimo Porta, Alison R. Bishop and Eva M. Kohner

Diabetic Retinopathy Unit, Dept. Medicine, Royal Postgraduate Medical School, Du Cane Road, London W12 0NN, UK.

Achieving and maintaining the best possible metabolic control is an important goal for diabetic patients, which should be pursued with the highest determination by their doctors and nurses. Success in this quest also requires much determination on the part of the patient, as it involves a number of procedures ranging from home monitoring of blood glucose during the day to self delivery of insulin throughout their entire life. While this may become a burden for the less than dedicated patient, it may be virtually impossible for diabetic people with visual problems to cope with the manual procedures involved in the self management of their condition. It may be argued that the whole purpose of maintaining optimal metabolic control, ie the prevention of ophthalmological and other chronic complications of diabetes, has already been lost in those patients who have low vision or are totally blind. However, even in these cases, good metabolic balance may still offer many benefits, both in terms of reducing the risk of neuropathic complications, ulcers and limb amputations and possibly, from a psychological point of view, in making the patient feel that he/she is not a "lost cause" and that self management of diabetes should continue as actively as possible. Over recent years this ambitious goal has been made attainable by the development of aids that can help patients with poor vision or even legal blindness to cope with such tasks as selecting and injecting the right quantity of insulin, mixing different insulin preparations in the same syringe and self-monitoring of their own blood sugar.

Devices for the Injection of Insulin

Inserting a syringe needle into the rubber cap of an insulin vial and then drawing the correct amount of insulin into the syringe are critical steps in the day to day management of diabetes. These apparently simple procedures mean, for a patient with low vision, total dependence on another person to carry out the tasks on his/her behalf. Answers to these problems range from simple but clever practical aids to sophisticated developments of the syringe as we know it in its traditional form. The occasional help of a person with good sight may or may not still be required. Appropriately moulded plastic trays are available that will accommodate the insulin vial on one side and the syringe on the other, thus providing a secure guide to facilitate accurate piercing of the top (Hypoguard Woodbridge, Suffolk, UK). The same manufacturer also produces a metal funnel that helps in guiding the needle into the insulin bottle.

The simplest way to draw up the correct amount of insulin is to cut a notch on the plunger of a plastic syringe so that it can be felt by the visually handicapped patient, indicating to him/her when the plunger has been properly withdrawn. An additional notch can be cut on the plunger if a second insulin preparation is to be mixed with the first. Two different vials of insulin can be made recognisable by a colour code or, in the case of total blindness, by sticking a piece of elastoplast around one of the two bottles of insulin. One manufacturer provides touch-coded caps on some insulin preparations (Novo Nordisk, Copenhagen, Denmark). Obviously, all these procedures must be carried out in advance by a person with normal vision (Jones *et al.*, 1989).

Another inexpensive solution is provided by a disposable tongue depressor. These are usually thin wooden sticks at the centre of which a slit can be cut to accommodate one wing of the syringe. The piston of the syringe can be pulled up to the desired dose of insulin and the stick is then cut across at the point reached by the external extremity of the piston. The patient can insert the syringe needle into the insulin vial and then, holding the vial in the uppermost position, withdraw the piston until it reaches the cut edge of the wooden stick, thus knowing that the correct amount of insulin has been drawn up. If a second insulin preparation is to be mixed with the first, then a second wooden stick is cut to the appropriate length and the two sticks can be attached to each other so that the slits are at the same level and the patient uses them for each specific insulin (Ravina, 1989). A commercial elaboration on the above is constituted by plastic syringe guides manufactured by Terumo (Brussels, Belgium) and Becton-Dickinson (Oxford, UK). This system requires the initial intervention of a person with good vision to cut the sticks at the correct length.

Patients with poor vision but not totally blind can obtain great help simply by using specially designed magnifiers that can be adapted to insulin syringes. These can click onto the insulin vial at one end and onto the syringe at the other end and magnify the length of the syringe scale or part of it. They are marketed by at least three different firms (Becton-Dickinson, Hypoguard, Monoject-Sherwood, London, UK).

Regular plastic insulin syringes can also be used in a gadget that permits blind or poorly sighted individuals to fill their own syringes with more than one insulin preparation. This machine (Count-a-Dose, Medistron, Horsham, West Sussex, UK) is fitted with a thumb wheel that enables the user to hear and feel how much insulin is being drawn up as each click represents 2 units of insulin. Two bottles of different insulins can be held at the other end, thus enabling safe and accurate dosage of the hormone.

All the above methods make use of commonly available plastic syringes which do not require particular modifications. Specially designed syringes, however, have been marketed for use by visually handicapped people with diabetes. One such syringe is the 'Click-count' model manufactured by Hypoguard. This is a glass 1 ml syringe that enables insulin to be drawn up by sound and touch. The plunger is turned by 90 degrees and the insulin drawn up with each 2 units being represented by a click. Turning the plunger back allows the injection to be given smoothly. This syringe offers flexibility in that it allows for mixed doses of different insulins to be drawn up, but one problem associated with the device is that some patients find it heavy and the plunger difficult to rotate into the drawing up and injecting modes.

The 'Preset' syringe manufactured by Rand Rocket, (Durham, UK) is slightly more complicated and requires a sighted person to set two screws attached to the plunger, which has a thread down its length. The screws are set at the appropriate length of the plunger and insulin can be drawn up until the screws prevent further movement. An additional shortcoming of this syringe is that only one type of insulin can be used.

A problem common to all the devices described so far is linked to the patients' inability to detect the presence of air in the syringe. This may be of minor importance in the case of a single air bubble, although even this may reduce the total dose of insulin delivered by 2–4 units, but becomes a major concern if the vial is empty or half empty with the patient unable to realise that too little or no insulin is actually drawn up and injected. Such risks can be minimised by advising the patient to:

1. Draw insulin into the syringe once, only to wet the barrel, needle and dead space, and then push it back into the vial; this should ensure that air bubbles will be pushed into the vial and smaller ones, or none at all, will form when the hormone solution is drawn up a second time;
2. Always draw up insulin very slowly;
3. Always keep the vial above the syringe so that the needle is totally immersed in the liquid;
4. Start a new vial if unsure of how much insulin is left, then ask a sighted person (when possible) whether it is safe to keep using the old one.

The problem of air bubbles is now superseded by the new concept of portable insulin syringe, pioneered by John Ireland 10 years ago (Paton *et al.*, 1981) and elaborated into the NovoPen series (Novo Nordisk). The first NovoPen resembles a fountain pen, in which the ink tank is replaced by an insulin cartridge and the nib is replaced by the needle. When the cap is removed and placed at the other end of the pen, it becomes a plunger. Each depression of this plunger pushes 2 units of insulin through the needle. This type of pen injector totally eliminates the need to draw insulin up from the insulin vial and is very easy to use, both for normal sighted patients and for those with low or no vision. The main limitation of this NovoPen is that the patient may miscount the number of depressions, especially if the amount of insulin required is high. The evolution of NovoPen I into NovoPen II has overcome this problem as it delivers the whole dose with just one depression of the plunger. A dialling system makes a clicking sound every two units, so that the total amount being drawn up is counted easily, both by touch and sound. The dial can be returned to zero if the patient has lost count of the number of clicks. In addition, a locking device has to be operated when insulin has been loaded, before the injection can be given. A great variety of cartridges are now available offering short and longer acting insulins.

A good compromise between the ingenious, but more expensive Pen injectors and the traditional insulin syringe remains the original Penject system now manufactured by Hypoguard (Paton *et al.,* 1981). A normal insulin syringe is filled completely by a sighted person and then fitted into the Penject system. This can then be left with the patient who can select the right amount of insulin to be delivered by the usual dialling click system. The autonomy allowed depends on the insulin requirement of each individual patient, although more syringes can be prepared in advance and kept in the refrigerator for several days.

Aids to Self-Monitoring of Blood Glucose

The simplest way of self-monitoring metabolic control is regularly checking urine for glycosuria. A meter for use with urine reagent strips is available for patients with low vision, and communicates the results by buzzing them as a code (Hypo-test Audio Urine Test Meter, Hypoguard). Testing of urine, however, is not the best way of assessing blood glucose control as glycosuria may depend on the individual renal threshold and does not pick up rapid variations of blood glucose concentration in insulin requiring patients. However, it remains an acceptable option for most subjects with stable, well controlled non-insulin dependent diabetes.

Self-monitoring of blood glucose provides more precise information but is definitely more complicated and can prove cumbersome even for normally sighted people. It requires a skilled and often painful pricking of the finger tip by blood letting lancets, the collection of a neat drop of blood onto the tiny reactive area of a blood glucose testing strip and correct placement of the latter in the slot of a meter. Every step of this procedure has to be timed precisely. Correct contact of blood with the reagent strip can be facilitated by a strip guide which has recently been made available by Hypoguard. This includes a chamber into which the blood is sucked by capillarity and comes into contact with the appropriate part of the reagent strip when the latter is pulled out of the device itself. The procedure also ensures that correct wiping of the strip is carried out by the gadget itself. This system, as well as being very practical, has been shown to improve the accuracy and reliability of blood glucose readings based on reflectance meters even in the hands of paramedical personnel in hospital wards (Rayman and Day, 1988).

Once the glucose reagent strip has been properly treated with blood, a number of glucose meters are available that have been designed for patients with low vision. The standard Hypocount B model has a large LED display so that partially sighted people can often manage adequately with it. The Hypocount B can be equipped either with a buzzing display that communicates the results by a code of sounds or with a built-in voice synthesizer that announces the reading directly to the patient, in addition to the visual display. All these devices are designed by Hypoguard and are for use with Boehringer reagent strips (Mannheim, FRG).

The Audio Glucocheck 90 (Medistron) gives the results by visual display, as well as by a series of bleeps and also a musical code warning if the reading was too high or too low. This machine has the additional advantage of using all major reagent strips.

Evaluation of the Techniques

There are hardly any published reports in which the above techniques have been evaluated for their efficiency, advantages and drawbacks. Consequently, most comments are based upon first hand experience, albeit limited to a few patients for each particular device. The NovoPen I was studied in this unit in a group of visually handicapped diabetic patients and found to improve metabolic control slightly, but significantly over 6 months (Hyer et al., 1988). All of 12 patients were assessed by questionnaire and appreciated the flexibility of meal times allowed by multiple injections of soluble insulin. Seven felt more relaxed and six felt they had become more active. A similar study is currently being carried out on the NovoPen II, to assess the potential additional advantages of delivering other available insulin formulations (ie a mixture of rapid and intermediate) by this device.

There are, however, practical problems which make it difficult to evaluate objectively most available aids for visually handicapped patients. Although diabetes remains an important cause of blindness early detection of diabetic retinopathy and its treatment by photocoagulation are reducing the number of patients with severe visual impairment. Thus, individual clinics may find it difficult to recruit sufficient individuals to carry out properly controlled studies.

Another question is whether the potentially increased independence achieved through some of the devices described represents a real advantage, as some of the patients may wish to maintain the company and support of somebody who visits them daily to measure and inject their insulin. On the other hand, much emphasis is being placed nowadays on the desirability of diabetic patients being independent of third parties for such vital manouvers (Assal et al., 1985). The helper, whether the District Nurse or a relative, may be unable to attend, perhaps at no notice and for reasons beyond control, leaving the visually handicapped diabetic patient at risk, helpless and under stress. Furthermore, all the persons interviewed in this unit before and after treatment with the NovoPen I appreciated the increased flexibility at mealtimes and 7 out of 12 felt more relaxed about their diabetes (Hyer *et al.*, 1988). Home monitoring of blood glucose is mostly carried out by pregnant and young insulin-dependent individuals but has proven valuable in improving metabolic control also in elderly patients (Martin *et al.*, 1986). However, for reasons supposedly similar to those outlined above, no trials have been published on the possible effectiveness of self-monitoring in the visually handicapped. One can presume that it would be useful for these patients to be able to check their own blood glucose if and when they feel unwell. In selected cases proper self monitoring might be psychologically rewarding.

Summary and Conclusions

Loss of vision is a devastating experience that is likely to increase the fears of diabetic patients for their own health, their dependence on third parties for simple tasks like insulin delivery and checking their own metabolic status and stimulate concerns over how to cope should any emergency arise and how to prevent such emergencies. Education has proved paramount in reducing the incidence of long term complications of diabetes, in particular foot ulcers and limb amputations, by obtaining the patients' informed collaboration in the maintenance of the best possible control (Assal *et al.*, 1985). Teaching the correct techniques for self-delivery of insulin and self-monitoring may prove extremely difficult in visually handicapped patients, as a lengthy personalised process of trial and error exercises is required to master techniques that even normally sighted individuals may find demanding and unpleasant. On the other hand, achieving these skills is particularly rewarding to both educators and patients, and a range of products are now available to facilitate their task. If these do not help to eliminate blindness, they can reduce some causes of distress caused by it and improve the patients' self-confidence and ability to live with their disease.

References

Assal, P., Mulhauser, I., Pernet, A., Gfeller, R., Jorgens, V. and Berger, M. (1985). Patient education as the basis for diabetes care in clinical practice and research. *Diabetologia* **28**, 602–613.

Hyer, S.L., Froyd, H.E. and Kohner, E.M. (1988). Effect of the NovoPen on glycaemic control and patient independence in diabetics with visual impairment. *Diabetic Medicine* **5**, 107–109

Jones, J.N. and Uccellari, H. (1989) *Coping with visual loss*. British Diabetic Association, London, pp 1–20.

Martin, B.J., Young, R.E. and Kesson, C.H. (1986). Home monitoring of blood glucose in elderly non-insulin dependent diabetics. *Practical Diabetes* **3**, 37.

Paton, J.S., Wilson, M., Ireland, J.T. and Reith, S. (1981). Convenient pocket insulin

syringe. *Lancet* **1**, 189–90.
Ravina, A. (1989). A Simple insulin-dosing device for diabetics with impaired vision. *Medicographia* **11** (suppl 1) 87.
Rayman, G. and Day, J.L. (1988). New device to improve the accuracy of bedside blood glucose tests. *Lancet* **2**, 1107–1109.

Explaining and Expanding the Role of the Chiropodist in the Care of People with Diabetes

Christopher Stiles

East Dorset Health Authority, Community Services Unit, Shaftesbury Road, Poole, Dorset BH15 2NT, UK.

Chiropody does not rely routinely upon high technology to perform its primary function of preventing, treating, and where possible curing the foot lesions of patients with diabetes. In the research field, technology may well aid the diagnosis and assist with evaluation of new techniques which are being developed to correct the effects of neuropathic ischaemic diabetic ulceration. Advanced techniques, manual skills, and the ability to apply academic concepts to patient care are the mainstay of the chiropodist and it is in this area that they provide the greatest benefit to the patient and provide maximum support in the team approach to the care of the person with diabetes.

Total Contact Casting

The development of new, light weight splinting material has enabled the chiropodist to develop methods of immobilising certain types of diabetic ulcer without the utilisation of costly hospital beds or the cost to the patient of becoming immobile either at home or as an inpatient on the ward. A variety of total contact casts have been developed from the Scotch Cast boot. Some are worn at all times encasing the leg and foot, others are detachable providing support during the day. All have been shown to be effective where the design criteria and patient selection models have been strictly adhered to. The technique requires a high degree of skill from the Chiropodist who alone, or if available, in conjunction with plaster technicians, applies the cast material to the patients leg. It is essential that the correct pressure is applied to ensure the efficiency of the cast. Prior to the application of the cast an exhaustive clinical assessment has taken place in collaboration with the diabetologist and where appropriate the members of the surgical team. Once the decision has been made to cast as an alternative to immobilisation or bed rest, a detailed educational programme is offered to the patients so that they will understand the process and the outcome. Their co-operation and trust is vital if the procedure is to work. Prior to the application of the cast a contract is formed between patient and practitioner based upon understanding of the outcome, the possible risks and the alternatives. The lynchpin of the contract is trust and informed consent. The cost benefit to the patient and to the hospital cannot be overlooked.Patients can continue with their daily living with only limited inconvenience. They do not lose money through not working or being hospitalised. The cast provides a symbol which allows patients to accept an otherwise unpleasant condition since, unlike a bandage, no exudate is visable. The plaster confirms the serious nature of the condition and legitimises the patients, status in the eyes of their peer group. Expensive bed time is not taken up by otherwise well people who, prior to the introduction of antibiotics and new techniques in diabetic ulcer control, might well have occupied a bed for up to six weeks, during which time they may have required skin grafting or resection of underlying boney structures.

Total contact casting is one of a number of preventative techniques used to heal diabetic ulcers. These techniques together with the use of antibiotic therapy and a high level of patient education has contributed to the reduction of amputation in the patient with diabetes. Various assessments of the decrease in below knee amputation have been made and these range from 30% to 47% reported by Davidson (1983). Connor (1987) in his chapter "The economic impact of diabetic foot disease" put the cost of a below knee amputation in 1982 at £8,500. This total did not take into account the cost to the patient in monetary and/or quality of life terms or to the external agencies involved in the rehabilitation and maintenance of the amputee.

Hill suggested..

"amputation as an end result of diabetic foot disease represents a failure in medical treatment. Many amputations could be avoided by patient education, a good chiropody service, and a good shoe fitting service. A failure to appreciate these simple facts results in amputation with its attendant cost and suffering. Resources used for patient education, chiropody services, and shoe fitting services prove very cost effective.

"The chiropodist working in the diabetic team has developed a high degree of specialisation and cost effectiveness since there is a positive cost benefit from using the chiropodist rather than taking up the more expensive and generalised skills of the houseman or registrar attached to the diabetic team." (Hill, 1987).

Surgical Intervention

Surgical intervention by the chiropodist may take a variety of forms. The main areas are the removal of either the whole or part of the nail under local analgesia, the debridement of neuropathic ischaemic ulcers and the removal of necrotic tissue, the removal of sequestrum from ulcerative sites over joints and the investigation of back-tracking sinuses for deep pockets of infection. The cost benefit of using a chiropodist for any or all of these procedures is obvious. In terms of skill mix it makes the most efficient use of the members of the diabetic care team since by freeing the medical members to undertake the tasks for which only they are qualified it provides a more systematic approach to the patients needs. The use of skill mix as a cost benefit to the health process is being addressed within the contex of the White Paper (H.M.S.O. 1989). Professional protectionism apart, there are many areas where highly skilled practitioners within the professions allied to medicine are well able to make a more positive contribution to patient care than has hitherto been perceived to be within their capabilities. Thus releasing both doctors and nures to perform other tasks for which they are trained.

Two areas of specialisation have so far been discussed but against this we have to look at the training, perceived role and position of the present day chiropodist within both the diabetic team and the public at large.

Chiropodial Training in the United Kingdom

Chiropody has evolved from the itinerent barber surgeon corn cutters who practised their art in fairgrounds, barber shops and the like through the transitional period of medical auxiliary to the current status of a profession allied to medicine. One of the most jealously guarded aspects of chiropodial training is the autonomy of the practitioner who has the right to accept patients formulate their treatment plans, undertake the treatment and discharge the patients without referral to any other agency.

New entrants into the schools of chiropody are required to have a minimum of two 'A' levels in appropriate scientific studies. They progress through three years of training which involves a carefully balanced mixture of academic, practical and clinical observation, increasing emphasis is placed upon the ability to make the quantum leap between the academic and the practical application of the acquired knowledge during this period of training. At the end of three years the new members of the profession leave with a diploma in podiatric medicine.

Chiropodists in the United Kingdom saw America as pointing the way to an improved scope of practice and enhanced professional recognition reversing the negative image currently held of chiropody by the population at large.

The Chiropodial Image

The confusing nature of training and the multiplicity of designatory letters following the name of chiropodists does little for the standing of the profession in the eyes of the general public. Because of the areas of practice within which chiropodists operate they do not achieve a high profile in the public eye. With the exception of the chiropody teams operating within the National Health Service most chiropodists work as individuals practising in isolated surgeries with little or no professional contact with their colleagues either within the profession or within the wider ambit of medical care. Less than 10% of the chiropodial workforce within the National Health Service are employed in hospital clinics and of these the vast majority would be involved in diabetic specialties. A report by the Royal College of Physicians and British Diabetic Association on the provision of diabetic services in 1984 indicated there was slightly less than one chiropodist per diabetic clinic in the United Kingdom. This did not take into account the fact that perhaps only 30% of all people with diabetes are routinely seen in hospital, the vast majority of care for diabetic patients is undertaken in the Community.

Chiropody lacks the charisma of nursing or medicine and is never the subject of media attention, nor do chiropodists appear as heroes and heroines in fictional roles. Professions develop strong images in the public mind. Professions like medicine which have a strong professional image well understood by the average person in the street can afford to be lampooned in comedy programmes like *Doctor in the House* or idealised in series like *Jimmies, Casualty*, and the forerunner of all medical programmes, *Dr. Kildare*. For the chiropodist no such strong role model exists with the exception of passing references to the chiropodist in the Archers. The only two programmes which have featured chiropodists in the last ten years have shown them as rather pathetic figures dealing either with a foot fettish or in an unsuccessful film attempt to kill a pig ("A private function").

The professional isolation and the lack of a high profile in the public eye ensures that the real value of the chiropodist is underestimated in health care terms and whilst reports on elderly care and on diabetes mentions the role of the chiropodist, no serious attempt has been made adequately to fund the provision of surgeries and staff within the hospital diabetic department. It is not unusual for the chiropodists "room" to be situated at some distance from the mainstream diabetic department which defeats the object of teamwork and cooperation. It is essential, if true cooperation and patient care is to be achieved, that the chiropodist, diabetologist and other members of the team work in close proximity so that any cross referrals which may become necessary during treatment may be carried out with the minimum of inconvenience to other members of the team and with maximum benefit to the patient. This is not achieved where the chiropodist operates at some distance from the diabetic department. It is unlikely that a busy consultant or registrar will have time to walk several hundred yards which may be required in some hospitals to span the distance between one consulting room and the other. The result is that patients may be required to make a separate appointment at the hospital another time or to seek help from their general practitioner which will require further time involvement in writing referral letters by the hospital team.

The Diabetic Team

Where teams exist it has been noted the paramedics are seen as peripheral to the main work of the diabetic department.

> "...the consultant asks the paramedical staff if they 'have anything'. Each in turn reports on what they see as any problems in dealing with patients from the day hospital who have been referred to them for physiotherapy or other services. For the most part this is an exercise in reporting. Each paramedical has a 'turn' and when this section of the meeting is over the chiropodist and physiotherapist also leave". (Smith and Cantley, 1985).

From this it may be concluded that the information derived from paramedics is of limited value to the diabetic team at large.

> "the paramedical staff are limited in their influence within a clearly defined organisational space. The chiropodist, for example, speaks only about the chiropodial aspects of patient care and then only when asked to do so. When the topic of chiropody is over, she leaves. In practice, here, teamwork means specialisation and the ready provision of a range of services to which patients can be referred by the sister and the consultant in charge." (Smith and Cantley, 1985).

When examining the literature on diabetes published in the United Kingdom mixed perceptions of the role of the chiropodist can be found. Faris (1982) sees the chiropodist "as an essential member of the team which cares for people with diabetes and who takes a major responsibility for the provision of this advice and support". At the other end of the spectrum the chiropodist is referred to as a toenail trimmer and callus pairer (Boulton *et al.*, 1990). A more positive view of the role of the chiropodist is taken in the report on the provision of medical care for adults with diabetes in the United Kingdom where close liaison with chiropody services, vascular surgeons and orthopaedic surgeons is seen to be necessary for the wellbeing of all diabetic patients. One of the recommendations in the report was that "a chiropodist should be present at every diabetic clinic as facilities for the prevention and treatment of foot ulceration are essential" (Royal College of Physicians and British Diabetic Association, 1984).

In contrast to the United Kingdom literature, in America the podiatrist is featured widely in the provision of care for patients with diabetes. Frykbert (1982) wrote that "The podiatrist specialising only in the care of the foot has correspondingly assumed an integral role in the management of the diabetic patient." Frykbert went on to outline the kind of cooperation which is required to ensure total care for the patient whilst indicating areas where routine care is undertaken.

"... 'bathroom surgery' and self treatment or neglect of such relatively minor disorders frequently lead to the more serious consequences of infection ulceration and gangrene. The podiatrist is often the first physician to discover or treat these disorders and it is imperative at this point to coordinate his efforts with those of the internist to ensure proper overall care of the patient." (Frykbert, 1982)

When comparing the literature on foot care in diabetes mellitus between United Kingdom and America it becomes increasingly obvious that the question of cost effectiveness is more strongly entrenched in the American idiology than has been seen in the medical establishment in the United Kingdom until the recent impact of the White Paper (H.M.S.O., 1989).

The Potential Role of Chiropodists in the Provision of Care for Patients with Diabetes

Much emphasis has been made on the provision of diabetic care within the hospital setting but it must be understood that only some 30% of all diabetic patients attend hospital routinely and of these perhaps only some 20% will present as at risk from neuropathic ischaemic ulceration. It follows therefore that the majority of patients with diabetes will present either in private practice or in the National Health Service Community Chiropody clinics established throughout the United Kingdom. It is in these clinics that the standard of care whilst universally high, suffers from the lack of provision of both staff and resources to enable the patient with diabetes to receive the amount of time which they may require for the maintenance of their chiropodial condition. In a busy community clinic where the majority of the patients are elderly, the inclusion of high risk diabetic patients whose treatment regimen may require weekly visits, presents an unreasonable demand upon an already overstrained service.

In future development of chiropody services for patients with diabetes it is essential that provision both in terms of staffing and finances be made available to ensure that mini clinics dealing exclusively with the needs of diabetic patients be developed within the community setting linked with the evolving mini clinics run by many G.P. group practices. It is essential to establish the autonomy of these clinics to ensure that they do not become a mere clearing ground for the general practice which they serve. As with their hospital colleagues, they should be seen as partners in diabetic care rather than providers of a second rate service based on want rather than need.

Collaborative studies between physicians researching diabetic foot care and chiropodists are rare outside teaching hospitals and it is only in the last two years that a chiropody department has been involved to any great extent in a community study on the problems of the diabetic foot.

Cost benefits always feature high on the agenda and in a study on technology and outpatient review, primary evaluation of the podiatric and chiroporactic treatments was included looking specifically at medical case management for high cost patients as a means of developing a cost containment strategy.

> "This service is targeted to the small proportion of the population that accounts for a large share of health resources: utilisation and cost analysis consistently find that as few as 10% of a given group consume up to 70% of the total health care expenditures." (Bergman *et al.*, 1990).

It is significant that in a country providing predominantly private and insurance funded health care the cost benefit implications of chiropody/podiatry should be of prime importance in the delivery of care. In the United Kingdom as the result of the fundamental changes in the Health Service in "Working for Patients" (H.M.S.O., 1989) that it is only now that the providers of care and the purchasers of care are coming together to examine in detail the cost of providing adequate care to patient groups.

New methods of treatment for patients with diabetic neuropathic ulceration have led to the reduction in amputations by as much as 50% and the length of stay in hospital by 85% (Davidson, 1983: Miller *et al.*, 1981 cited by Hill, 1987).

The Expanding Role of the Chiropodist

I have concentrated on the current role of the chiropodist but there is an expanding role which needs to be recognised and which has been under-utilised in the provision of chiropody services. The chiropodist is uniquely placed in the clinical situation to listen to the patient and, by skillful questioning, is able to elicit much information which, because of time constraints, it is not available to the physician. It is this aspect of the chiropodial service which is vastly under-used. In a busy outpatient department it is rare for the consultant to spend an extended amount of time upon patient enquiry. Throughput pressures preclude protracted conversations. It is for those fortunate few patients who have foot pathologies requiring the attention of the chiropodist that a listening board is provided. The chiropodist, whilst delivering care and education to the patient, is also able to assimilate background information and symptoms which may not, to the patient, appear significant enough to 'bother' the consultant with. In a well designed diabetic department the chiropodist has a surgery adjacent to the consultant's suite and when information which requires action is illicited from the patient it is possible for the consultant or registrar to be consulted rapidly and for the patient to be examined without taking up much valuable consultant time. It may well be that an infection has been discovered that requires antibiotic cover and there is a clear benefit to the patient obtaining a prescription at once rather than having to go to their own G.P. or having to return to the hospital.

Chiropody and chiropodists are increasingly involved in the provision of preventative education for patients with diabetes and they have become an essential part of the educational team. It has been demonstrated that the most efficient use of the educational session by chiropodial staff is to provide an informal discussion and information session followed by an individual assessment of each new patient who is accepted into the hospital programme. By this means both the counselling and the clinical skills of the chiropodist can be employed at their most effective and, as I have indicated above, they can operate as an information filter to the consultant who is managing the overall care of the patient with diabetes.

Summary and Conclusions

In conclusion, by providing adequate funding and recognition for the expanding role of the chiropodist in the diabetic care team, considerable cost benefits and advantages may be gained by the patient, the reduction in below knee amputations and hence the reduction in mortality rates following this procedure would amply justify the resulting funding which will be required to implement the requirements of the new chiropody services. It cannot be emphasised strongly enough that the chiropodist is seen as part of the diabetic team and does not claim ascendancy over any other member but rather seeks the recognition which, for the reasons which I have outlined above, has been denied to the profession in the United Kingdom (Davidson, 1983).

References

Bergman, A, Henderson, B, and Cline, J L, (1990) Technology and outpatient review: a preliminary evaluation *Quality Review Bulletin* **16**, 234–239
Boulton, A (1990) The diabetic foot, pp.293–306 In Tattersall R and Gale E A M (eds) *Management of Diabetes Mellitus* London: Churchill Livingstone
Connor, H (1987) The economic impact of diabetic foot disease, pp.145–149.Connor, H, Boulton, A J M, Ward, J D (eds) *The foot in diabetes* London: John Wiley and Sons
Davidson, JK (1983) The Grady Memorial Hospital Diabetes Unit Ambulatory Care Programme *Exerpta Medica International Congress Series* No 642 pp 286–97
Faris, I (1982) *The management of the diabetic foot* New York: Churchill Livingstone
Frykbert, RG (1982) Padiatric practice in diabetes. In Kozak, GP (ed) *Clinical Diabetes Mellitus,* W B Saunders: Philadelphia
H.M.S.O. (1989) *Working for Patients.* London: H.M.S.O.
Hill, R D (1987) *Diabetes health care* London: Chapman and Hall
Royal College of Physicians and British Diabetic Association (1984) Joint Report. *The Provision of Medical Care for Adult Diabetic Patients in the United Kingdom in 1984.* London: British Diabetic Association
Smith, G and Cantley, C (1985) *Assessing Health Care.* Milton Keynes: Open University Press

Psychological Aspects of the Diabetes Control and Complications Trial

John R. Kramer, Alan M. Jacobson, Christopher M. Ryan, William D. Murphy, and the DCCT Research Group

The DCCT Research Group, Box NDIC/DCCT, Bethesda, MD 20892, USA.

This chapter will focus on the psychological ramifications of a long-term treatment study, the Diabetes Control and Complications Trial (DCCT). The DCCT will be described, followed by a discussion of three major issues: (a) selection of psychological endpoints (b) screening of study applicants and (c) patient management during the trial. While every clinical trial is in certain respects unique, it is hoped that lessons learned from the DCCT will be relevant to other large-scale diabetes treatment studies.

Overview of the Study

The DCCT is a randomized, controlled trial of the effects of intensive diabetes therapy on the development and progression of complications among individuals with insulin-dependent (Type I) diabetes mellitus (DCCT, 1990). The study's purpose is to determine whether keeping blood glucose values close to those of individuals without diabetes will reduce the appearance and/or progression of microvascular complications. Retinopathy is the primary endpoint, with nephropathy, neuropathy, and cardiovascular disease also being studied. In addition to any benefits of intensive versus standard therapy, the DCCT is studying the relative risks and costs of the two treatment regimens.

The overall study is divided into a primary prevention trial and a secondary intervention trial. The first addresses the question of whether intensive treatment will prevent or delay the appearance of complications in subjects who exhibit no evidence of retinopathy at study onset. The second addresses the question of whether intensive treatment will affect the progression of complications in subjects who exhibit early signs of retinopathy at baseline. A total of 1,441 subjects with insulin-dependent diabetes, aged 13–39 (726 primary prevention and 715 secondary intervention subjects) have been randomly assigned to receive either standard therapy or experimental intensive therapy at one of 29 clinics in the United States and Canada.

The major goal of the experimental treatment regimen is to maintain glycemic control similar to individuals without diabetes. Preprandial blood glucose levels of 70–120 mg./dL and postprandial levels less than 180, determined with self-monitoring, and glycosolated hemoglobin (HbA_{1c}) levels in the normal range have been established as the goals for this group. In addition, because of concern regarding nocturnal hypoglycemia, a weekly 3 a.m. blood glucose test is performed and therapy is adjusted if the level is not > 65 mg/dL. To achieve these goals, individuals in the experimental group receive three or more injections of insulin daily or subcutaneous insulin from a pump worn externally. Blood glucose level, diet, and exercise are taken into account when calculating insulin doses. Experimental group patients attend their DCCT clinic monthly, where blood is drawn for the HbA_{1c} assay and physicians, nurses, dietitians, and mental health professionals are consulted to assist with their regimen. In between clinic visits, participants are contacted by telephone to monitor daily blood glucose values and provide advice.

Standard treatment is designed to mimic conventional management of Type I diabetes, with one or two daily injections of insulin, self monitoring of urine or blood glucose, and diet instruction. Clinical well-being with no symptoms of hyper- or hypoglycemia is the clinical goal. Unlike the experimental regimen, blood or urine test results are not used to adjust insulin on a day-by-day basis in the absence of symptoms of hyper- or hypoglycemia. Subjects in the standard group visit their DCCT clinic every three months, where blood is collected for the measurement of HbA_{1c} and physicians, nurses, dietitians, and mental health professionals are available for routine follow-up care.

The DCCT was initially conceived and planned in 1982–1983 (Phase I; DCCT, 1986). A feasibility study of the first 278 subjects was conducted in 1984–1985 (Phase II; DCCT, 1987). The trial itself is now more than halfway through its projected course (Phase III; 1985–1993; DCCT; 1990). Sample size and trial duration have been chosen so that during Phase IV, when data are analyzed, there will be more than a 90 percent chance of detecting a 33 percent difference in the treatment groups' rates of retinopathy development and progression (DCCT, 1988a). By virtue of its statistical power and prospective design, the DCCT represents the most systematic attempt ever to examine the effect of tight control on the development of complications in Type I diabetes (DCCT, 1988b).

It is anticipated that subjects will participate in the DCCT for 5 to 10 years. The trial's length and intense experimental regimen pose critical challenges to the maintenance of both patient and staff adherence. Moreover, any differential effects of the treatment regimens on psychological or neurobehavioral functioning or on quality of life are potentially important study outcomes. Many of these concerns, voiced at the DCCT's inception, are reflected in its screening and treatment procedures. As the study has unfolded over the past seven years, other psychological issues have surfaced. It is to such issues, both anticipated and revealed, that this chapter now turns. Since the investigators are masked to outcome data until study's end (an independent, external review group examines the data frequently), this chapter is descriptive in nature.

The Selection of Psychological Endpoints

Because diabetes and its treatment can have adverse psychological effects (e.g., Ryan, 1988; Jacobson, 1986), the DCCT established a system of periodically monitoring the psychological and cognitive functioning of patients during their participation in the trial. This constituted one component of a cost-benefit analysis in which potential benefits of treatment would be compared with its costs, as measured by time, effort, and possible physical or psychological sequelae.

During Phase I, a subcommittee was charged with identifying specific psychological domains considered to be most at risk in experimental treatment, as well as selecting or developing the instruments to measure, on a routine and systematic basis, functioning in these areas. Three major areas were delineated: (a) neurobehavioral functioning (b) psychiatric distress and (c) quality of life. For each domain, it was necessary to strike a balance between instruments that were highly labor- and time-intensive and measures that were too brief to provide meaningful information. In some instances, already published measures were incorporated; in other cases, instruments were created or modified expressly for the purposes of the DCCT.

Neurobehavioral Functioning

This area was targeted because a number of clinical studies suggested an association between Type I diabetes and the occurrence of electro-physiological (Eeg-Olofsson, 1977) and neuropsychological (Ryan, 1988) abnormalities in children and adults. Both very high, as well as very low, glucose levels are thought to be responsible for the development of these central nervous system changes (for review, see Ryan, 1990).

The majority of earlier studies were ill-equipped to answer etiological questions because of their cross-sectional and retrospective nature. In contrast, the DCCT's prospective, multifactorial design allows one to document the development of neurobehavioral deficits over several years and to examine their onset in relationship to physiological, demographic, and treatment parameters. If either treatment results in better (or worse) cognitive function, the study is equipped to identify such differences over time. Beyond this research issue, however, the battery serves the vital function of monitoring the individual patient's cognitive integrity and ensures that if either treatment is associated with an increase in morbidity, as signaled by a significantly higher rate of cognitive impairment, the study will be able to detect and address such an effect.

A three-to-four-hour battery of well-known, standardized neuropsychological tests is used to sample cognitive functions in a comprehensive fashion. Eight general cognitive domains are evaluated: general intellectual functioning; verbal skills; problem-solving and abstract reasoning; calculation skills; learning and memory; visuoperceptual and visuomotor skills; attention and perceptual motor skills; and motor speed and manual dexterity.

The battery was administered to subjects when they first entered the trial in order to establish baseline functioning. Subjects are reassessed during their second, fifth, and seventh year of participation, as well as at study termination. Trained neurobehavioralists administer the battery at each clinic. Scoring, coding, and interpretation are performed centrally. Each protocol is reviewed for possible changes from baseline performance. If evidence of clinically significant deterioration is found, the local clinic is alerted and further appropriate neurologic and psychological assessments are conducted. A more complete description of this process can be found elsewhere (Ryan *et al.*, in press).

Psychiatric Status

A second area of potential impact identified during the feasibility phase was psychological distress. At that time, few data were available regarding the long-term effects on psychiatric health of an intensive diabetes regimen. It was hypothesized that the greater demands of experimental treatment might cause subjects in that group to experience more distress than subjects in standard treatment. Several measures of psychiatric status were considered, including inventories designed to detect the presence of formal psychiatric disorders. This approach was not incorporated, primarily because there was no compelling theoretical or empirical reason to expect a greater incidence of actual psychiatric illness among experimental group subjects. In addition, the time and expense required to administer such inventories would be prohibitive. Instead, an economical but well-standardized measure of psychiatric status, the Symptom Check List (SCL-90-R), was chosen (Derogatis *et al.*, 1977).

The SCL-90-R is administered to all DCCT participants on an annual basis and consists of 90 self-rated symptoms that cover the past week (e.g. "How much were you distressed by feeling that most people cannot be trusted?"). Answers can be scored in terms of overall psychiatric distress (Global Severity Index; Positive Symptom Distress Index; Positive Symptom Total), or with respect to nine symptom dimensions which tap more specific aspects of distress: Somatization; Obsessive-Compulsive; Interpersonal Sensitivity; Depression; Anxiety; Hostility; Phobic Anxiety; Paranoid Ideation; and Psychoticism (Derogatis *et al.*, 1975). The two scoring systems enable the DCCT to determine whether experimental treatment causes an increase in overall psychiatric distress or along specific components thereof.

Quality of Life

An additional measure was sought to complement the psychiatric orientation of the SCL-90-R and describe participants' perceptions of well-being in relation to their illness. Careful consideration was given to existing functional health status measures (e.g., the Sickness Impact Profile of Bergner *et al.*, 1981) which had the advantage of standardization and an established research base. However, these instruments were deemed unsuitable for two reasons. First, they were targeted for patients who exhibit major restrictions of physical functioning, unlike DCCT participants who were free of such limitations at study outset and not likely to develop them over the course of the study. A second problem was that none of the health status instruments available at the time included items that address the impact of diabetes per se.

In response to this lack of diabetes-specific measures, the Diabetes Quality of Life Scale (DQOL) was developed for use in the trial (DCCT, 1988c). Items were based on the suggestions of patients, physicians, nurses, and mental health professionals. It was recognized that the final set of 46 multiple-choice questions could not measure all possible areas of patient concern or any single domain in great depth. Rather, an attempt was made to sample a wide range of experiences most likely to be affected by diabetes and its treatment.

The DQOL questions are pooled into four primary scales which address overlapping content areas from different perspectives. These include Satisfaction (e.g., "How satisfied are you with the amount of time it takes to manage your diabetes?"), Impact (e.g., "How often do you feel pain associated with the treatment for your diabetes?"), Diabetes Worry (e.g., "How often do you worry about whether you will pass out?"), and Social/Vocational Worry (e.g., "How often do you worry that because of your diabetes you are behind in terms of dating, going to parties, and keeping up with your friends?"). Worries were incorporated into the instrument because it was anticipated that study participation would cause patients to think more about their disease. A preliminary study of the measures' psychometric properties suggests it to have an acceptable degree of test-retest reliability, internal consistency, and construct and convergent validity (DCCT, 1988c). Although the DQOL was created for the DCCT, it transcends specific components of treatment (e.g., blood vs. urine testing; pumps vs. injections), and individuals with insulin-dependent diabetes in other settings may be able to use the scale as well.

Screening and Selection of Study Applicants

During Phase I, physicians, nurses, and mental health consultants (both within and outside the trial) participated in a series of meetings to design appropriate screening procedures. In addition to choosing candidates who met basic demographic (e.g., age) and physiological criteria (e.g., c-peptide secretion; DCCT, 1986; 1990) it was considered essential to select individuals who (a) were well-informed about, and appeared to understand, the trial's purpose and procedures and (b) were free of attributes that suggested major adherence problems.

A multimodal screening procedure was created to address these concerns (DCCT, 1989). Each applicant was evaluated for a period lasting several weeks to several months, which served the purpose of familiarizing a clinic with the candidate as well as educating the candidate comprehensively about the study. This extended interaction compensated for the fact that no single measure can accurately predict long-term compliance. Repeated exposure to the trial design and requirements thus maximized the likelihood of compliance by dissuading unsuitable candidates and preparing those who remained to the greatest degree possible.

Understanding and Expectations

Applicants who met demographic and physiological screening criteria were shown, with their families, a slide/tape show which provided an overview of the DCCT's purpose and design (DCCT, 1989). Throughout this presentation, questions were encouraged. Subjects who maintained interest in the study took home booklets which provided more detailed information about the trial. A quiz that focused on the study's purpose, procedures, and risks was then administered. Candidates were required to answer 90% of the items correctly. If they failed, they were asked to view the slide/tape show again or to review the study information booklet. An alternate version of the test was administered and the subject required to answer all questions correctly. Family members were also questioned about the study with structured interviews in order to ascertain that they understood the purposes, risks, and benefits of the DCCT.

These innovative educational strategies were, in our view, critical for ensuring that applicants had realistic expectations of the trial. It was assumed that such subjects would be less likely to have major problems with adherence or to become dissatisfied with the trial. Indeed, the atypically small number of dropouts and treatment crossovers (see "Overall Adherence and Satisfaction" below) provide strong support for the validity of this assumption.

Adherence

Few, if any, empirically validated predictors of adherence exist. One reason is the complexity of this concept. Viewed initially as a global, unitary patient characteristic, adherence is now recognized to involve a constellation of behaviors that are each influenced by environmental, cognitive, and affective variables (DiMatteo & DiNicola, 1982; Meichenbaum & Turk, 1987). Further, patients' levels of adherence to one component of a medical regimen generally do not predict their levels of adherence to other components; this holds true both across content domains (Orme and Binik, 1989) and within them (e.g., diet; Webb et al., 1984).

In light of the above considerations, we devised a set of screening procedures which targeted several facets of the diabetes regimen. A variety of approaches was employed, drawing on existing adherence theory and research.

Unilateral exclusion criteria

Because no reliable predictors of adherence were available, most screening measures were used to identify problems that warranted further inquiry before a final decision about a candidate could be made. A few criteria, however, automatically signaled exclusion: (a) a history of major psychiatric problems and/or substance abuse within the past five years (b) illiteracy (c) a strong indication that the subject could not perform the protocol or come to the clinic on a regular basis (d) any unresolvable objection to the study by a family member living with the applicant and/or (e) indications that the subject was following his or her current regimen very poorly (e.g., had at least 3 episodes of ketoacidosis in the past year).

The presence of any of the above conditions was considered sufficient to eliminate individuals from further consideration, in light of the emotional, intellectual, and behavioral demands of the protocol. It should be noted, however, that these data were gathered from structured interviews and tests designed for the DCCT and not from standardized, empirically established instruments. For this reason, caution was exercised in deciding whether, for example, an individual truly had experienced major depression. In such cases, conversations with family and appropriate community and mental health personnel were necessary to verify impressions gathered from screening.

Behavioral tasks

The screening process also incorporated two weeks of urine and blood testing, record keeping that included the times and results of these tests, and diaries of meals, exercise, and insulin regimens. The behavioral tasks provided subjects with a realistic approximation of experimental group treatment by engaging them in an intricate and demanding protocol. In addition, the tasks helped identify individuals who were at risk for adherence problems. Because an individual's behavior was viewed as a reasonable predictor of future similar behavior, subjects who did not perform the tasks well were viewed as poor candidates, particularly if additional training failed to correct matters. This process also allowed patients to make highly informed decisions about the likely degree of their satisfaction and compliance in the trial.

Applicant interviews

Structured interviews with the candidates constituted another component of screening. Applicants were asked about their availability for the study (e.g., "How flexible is your employer/school about giving you time off to keep doctor's appointments?"). They were also questioned about its benefits and drawbacks (e.g., "What do you think you will gain from the study?"; "What effect do you expect this study to have on your current daily routine?"). These topics were raised because adherence to treatment is influenced by patients' perceptions of its benefits and costs. According to the Health Belief Model, the more an individual views inconvenience, embarrassment, and other drawbacks as preeminent, the less fully he or she will comply with a protocol (Becker & Janz, 1985; Brownlee-Duffeck *et al.*, 1987).

The subject's willingness to be randomly assigned to treatment was a third area targeted by the interview (e.g., "Do you have a strong preference for being assigned to one treatment group over the other? If so, which do you prefer and why?"). It was considered important to screen out applicants who strongly preferred one treatment over the other, because adherence would suffer if patients were randomly assigned to treatment they perceived as less desirable (see chapter by Bradley in the final section of this book).

Family interviews

Significant family members were administered structured interviews that probed their knowledge of the DCCT (e.g., "Can you tell me what you understand to be the purpose of the DCCT?") and attitudes towards the study (e.g., "Would you be willing to support the decision of _____ to be randomized into either of the treatment groups"?) Emphasis was placed on family awareness of, and willingness to endure, drawbacks of the study such as distance, medical risks (e.g., hypoglycemic episodes), and time commitments. In essence, these questions served to measure social support, which correlates positively with patient adherence to medical regimens (e.g., Hauser *et al.*, 1990; Schlenk & Hart, 1984).

Self-predicted adherence

Another instrument employed for screening was the Request Behaviors Confidence Questionnaire, an outgrowth of self-efficacy research which suggests that people can accurately predict their probable levels of adherence (e.g., Bandura, 1989). The DCCT-created questionnaire contains 36 items on which applicants made numerical estimates of (a) their ability to carry out major components of the protocol (e.g., "How certain are you that you will be able to test your blood for glucose at 3:00 a.m. once a week?") and (b) the percentage of tasks they expected to perform (e.g., "If you are assigned to the experimental group, how often would you test your blood for glucose four times a day?"). Subjects completed the instrument both before and after performing the Behavioral Tasks in order to determine how well the second set of estimates corresponded with the actual two-week protocol for the tasks.

Patient Management During the Trial

Initial Results

The adherence of subjects selected for the trial has been recorded every three months during quarterly clinic examinations. Clinic staff complete forms that assess a patient's attendance, availability for phone calls, adherence to insulin algorithms and diet plan, and the timing, accuracy and completeness of blood or urine glucose tests. Satisfaction and psychiatric status have been measured through annual administrations of the DQOL and SCL-90-R, respectively (see "Quality of Life" and "Psychiatric Status" above).

Overall adherence and satisfaction

Although complete analyses of these data will not be conducted until the end of Phase III, the results available thus far suggest that subjects have complied well with the protocol. More than 95% of clinic appointments have taken place within the allotted time windows, and more than 95% of scheduled clinic lab tests have been completed. In the first year of the trial, between 81% and 84% of scheduled self-administered blood and urine glucose tests were reported by the subjects.

While information based on the DQOL and SCL-90 is not currently available, preliminary data suggest an unusually high level of patient satisfaction. Less than 1% of the 1,441 subjects are not participating currently, and less than 3% have switched from one treatment group to the other (DCCT, 1990). Such management crossovers are usually for a brief period of time, and we hope to maintain all subjects in their assigned groups.

Within these general indications of good adherence and satisfaction, there have been specific problems, stemming from the inherent frustrations of diabetes and from the rigorous requirements of experimental treatment. The following observations are impressions based on a) examination of individual patient records b) discussions with patients and staff at individual clinics c) discussions among staff at national meetings and d) review of this manuscript by all DCCT clinic mental health professionals. These observations, accumulated over the first seven years of the trial, do not spring from a systematic sampling of behavioral data. Nevertheless, considerable consensus exists regarding the major issues that are elaborated below. Some of them, particularly those dealing with prevalence (e.g., of weight gain and hypoglycemia), will be formally collated and analyzed at study's end. Other issues, particularly those dealing with patient motivations and feelings (e.g., about falsifying data) will remain impressions. None of the points presented below should be viewed as definitive at the present time.

Testing and timing

One major source of difficulty has been the need to test and record blood glucose levels at regular intervals. Most subjects in the experimental group appear to test the required 4 to 5 times per day, as suggested by the above statistics, but major lapses sometimes occur. The timing of tests and insulin has been more problematic. Participants report that frequently it is difficult to check their blood glucose and administer insulin 30 to 45 minutes before eating, particularly when they are busy or eating out.

The accuracy and completeness of self-administered glucose test results is a highly sensitive issue. It is our impression that many subjects have, at one time or another, deliberately reported data inaccurately, as suggested by (a) discrepancies between logbooks and electronic memories (Mazze, 1985) (b) patterns of deletions or manual insertions of values in the meter's memories and (c) blood glucose values that are markedly out of line with periodic laboratory profilset readings or HbA_{1c} values.

Based on discussions with participants, a number of psychological processes appear to contribute to this phenomenon. Some patients simply tire of study demands and present false readings to avoid discovery and confrontation over their reduced testing. The desire to please one's physician and nurse with good numbers is another factor. Self-esteem also plays a role; some participants find it difficult to admit to themselves or others that they have undesirable blood glucose readings. A fourth motive appears to be the frustration subjects report when they obtain high or low values that cannot be easily explained. The tediousness of trying to account for these occurrences to staff has caused some individuals to fabricate values that are within expected range.

Diet

The need to maintain a healthy diet and calculate food values accurately has been a constant challenge to study participants, particularly those in the experimental group. Although dietitians have carefully taught and regularly re-educated subjects to employ a diet consistent with American Diabetes Association guidelines, many participants report difficulties when eating out. The nutritional content of food consumed at relatives', friends', or restaurants can be difficult to estimate. Eating away from home also presents a timing problem because meal onset cannot always be predicted accurately.

Weight

Another area of difficulty has been weight gain. In the first year of the feasibility study (Phase II), experimental and standard group participants gained an average of 5.1 kg and 2.4 kg, respectively. Subjects whose HbA_{1c} levels decreased the most tended to gain the most, probably because of a reduction in glycosuria (DCCT, 1988d). At certain clinics, young female patients have admitted to binge eating and, in some cases, purging or reducing insulin in order to lose weight. Because systematic study-wide data are not available, it is not known what proportion of them meet formal diagnostic criteria for an eating disorder.

Unplanned eating also has contributed to weight problems. Snacking has sometimes been underestimated by patients, as revealed by discrepancies between their initial verbal estimates and subsequent written records.

Hypoglycemia

Insulin reactions have constituted a source of ongoing concern to both patients and staff. Despite overall reductions of 50% in the rate of severe hypoglycemia, experimental participants sustain severe reactions two to three times more often than do standard patients (DCCT, 1990). The majority of episodes occur during sleep or without warning when awake (Lorenz *et al.*, for the DCCT Research Group, 1988).

A second problem with hypoglycemia has been its effect on adherence to the experimental regimen. Participants describe themselves as fearful of reactions, embarrassed by them, and angry at the reduced mental efficiency that follows. It is not surprising that they try to avoid reactions, particularly before sleeping, engaging in high levels of activity, or operating machinery (e.g., automobiles). Strategies such as overeating or reducing insulin doses often result in blood glucose levels that exceed experimental treatment targets.

Maintaining Patient Well-Being, Satisfaction, and Adherence

The procedures employed to help sustain morale and performance represent a combination of mechanisms that were incorporated into the DCCT protocol at the beginning of the trial, as well as approaches that have been added over the past several years. Although impressions are positive and enthusiasm strong, no formal data are available as to the actual efficacy of these techniques, either singly or in combination.

Morale

Procedures to help maintain patient morale have stressed the study's importance and conveyed appreciation for the difficult task each participant faces. A national DCCT newsletter is distributed to all patients several times yearly with these messages. The director of the trial made a motivational videotape viewed by all participants, and he is currently visiting each center to meet patients personally. Certificates, gifts, and banquets have been used to reward continued participation in the study.

Well-being and adherence

The major mechanism established for optimizing well-being and adherence in experimental patients has been intensive contact and the consequent development of strong patient-provider and patient-patient bonds. A critical component of this process has been frequent telephone calls between experimental subjects and staff, most frequently the primary nurse. Phone calls have been used to identify problems, remind subjects to carry out specific assignments, collect data on these efforts, and provide verbal reinforcement.

Clinic events, held throughout the year, have often included patient support groups. These range from relatively unstructured sessions, where subjects provide each other comradeship and social support, to focused group discussions of topics such as stress management.

Individual and family counselling have assisted patients in confronting a wide range of personal and environmental obstacles to adherence. Because the need for therapy was anticipated, mental health professionals (psychologists, psychiatrists, social workers, and/or counselors) were assigned to each clinic. Although participants were screened to be free of major psychiatric disturbances, it was recognized that some of them would require therapeutic assistance over the course of the trial because of the stresses engendered by diabetes, the DCCT protocol, and other life circumstances not fully revealed during the screening period.

Participants with relatively circumscribed difficulties have been assisted by cognitive-behavioral techniques such as time management, relaxation training, assertion training, and behavioral contracts. The latter have been employed to combat problems with weight, testing, timing, and other components of the experimental regimen. Individuals suffering from more pervasive psychiatric problems have been treated with a spectrum of therapies based on cognitive, dynamic, and family process models. Certain therapeutic interventions, such as stress management, have sometimes improved metabolic control while also increasing patients' psychological well-being (e.g., Bradley, 1988).

Maintaining Staff Morale and Effectiveness

The DCCT experimental treatment regimen necessitates a high level of performance from providers as well as from patients. In their day-to-day efforts to encourage maximum patient compliance, clinic staff can become embroiled in numbers and lose sight of the study's primary purposes. In addition, the team approach sometimes blurs distinctions between disciplines. Procedures to resolve these dilemmas and foster professionals' effectiveness are described below. As with the techniques applied to patients, no systematic data exist on the efficacy of these approaches.

National meetings

All DCCT clinics and central administration meet three times yearly. Conferences provide collegial support as well as a forum for airing grievances and generating solutions. Physicians, nurses, mental health professionals, and nutritionists meet separately during part of these meetings, enabling them to address issues specific to their discipline as well as those that pertain to the study as a whole.

Adherence is invariably a major topic of discussion at national meetings, with presentations of particular cases or treatment approaches. Special meetings sometimes supplement the agenda. For example, an intensive two-day workshop was recently conducted by psychologists and dietitians to upgrade all dietitians' skills in interviewing, counselling, and behavior modification.

Clinic visits

A second major mechanism for maintaining staff morale and effectiveness has been the creation of "sister clinics." Each center that is doing relatively well in the study—in terms of morale, patient adherence, and glycemic control—has been assigned to a clinic that is not doing as well. Visits have been conducted between each pair of clinics, during which individual cases have been presented, as well as more general discussions of clinic organization and strategies. This one-on-one approach has been viewed as a useful supplement to the more generic information sharing and morale boosting that takes place at national meetings.

Mental health professionals

Psychologists, psychiatrists, social workers, and counselors have played a major role in facilitating staff well-being. Their efforts to improve its functioning have taken place at a number of levels, ranging from opinions expressed at clinic meetings to staff retreats, where problems with communication, organization, and the sharing of power have been discussed more intensively. Similar efforts have been exerted at national conferences, where mental health professionals have helped resolve differences and improve rapport between and within disciplines.

Lessons We Have Learned

Following is a summary of insights about patient management gathered from the first five years of the study. It is anticipated that more will surface with additional experience.

Staff-patient Relationships

The first five years of the DCCT have unveiled the complex nature of interactions between participants and staff. Many of the experimental subjects and clinic staff now know each other as well as close friends or family members. Such familiarity can generate emotional undertones that impede objective communication and treatment. For example, staff have at times blamed themselves for a subject's failure to comply or to control their HbA_{2c} levels. Conversely, some providers have interpreted a patient's lapses in adherence as a personal affront directed towards them. When asked to exert more effort, patients may feel "nagged" by staff in much the same way they feel admonished by a parent or spouse.

Staff-patient interactions are neither simple nor static. When a patient experiences a social or medical crisis, it is sometimes necessary to become highly directive, temporarily relinquishing the collaborative model that typifies routine interactions. Some participants tolerate these shifts well, while others resent the loss of autonomy and privacy that accompanies such changes.

Natural Contingencies

One of the most sobering realizations has been the potency of rewards and punishments over which staff have little control and which frequently sabotage our efforts to make behavioral changes. This dilemma is exemplified when a patient attempts to lower average blood glucose. Positive reinforcers provided by the clinic (e.g., praise, money, movie tickets) are often far less powerful than natural negative contingencies which may accompany such change. The latter may include weight gain, an increased incidence of insulin reactions, and the need for additional effort in record keeping, testing, timing, and diet.

The joint effect of these negative contingencies can be seen in experimental patients who achieve HbA_{1c} values that are below those at trial entry but remain significantly above the study goal. Such individuals often express satisfaction with their improved control but appear unwilling to lower their average blood glucose further.

In order to counteract these drawbacks, staff members have been forced to exercise considerable ingenuity. Few truly powerful reinforcers are at their disposal, particularly with regard to negative reinforcement and punishment. Ethical and scientific strictures do not allow subjects to be eliminated from the study or their medical care to be withheld. Thus, entreaties by staff for additional patient effort carry no ultimate threat in this regard. A number of clinics have asked participants to come to the clinic more often or stay overnight at the hospital when their glucose control has deteriorated beyond a preset level. In addition to providing useful diagnostic information to staff, such inconvenient and time-consuming visits also function as negative reinforcers. More frequent phone calls and additional record keeping are further examples of medically justifiable but unpleasant tactics that have in some cases motivated improvement through negative reinforcement.

Changes in Adherence and Control

When the DCCT was designed, the extent to which adherence might vary over time was not fully realized. Some subjects have improved dramatically over the course of the trial. Many adolescents, for example, were very non-compliant initially. They resented the restrictions imposed by diabetes and the DCCT, and they ignored much of the experimental regimen. As these subjects grew older, many of them began perceiving clinic staff as collaborators rather than extensions of their parents. Certain adolescents have taken more respons-ibility for their diabetes, with beneficial effects on adherence and glycemic control.

Other subjects have exhibited the reverse pattern, beginning their study participation at a high level of control and becoming increasingly careless with time. In some cases, boredom or "burnout" with the trial appear to have been primarily responsible. In other instances, life stresses, such as job loss or marital conflict, have been a major cause of this deterioration. Patients have admitted that the DCCT is less of a priority in their lives under such circumstances. As these stresses resolve, some participants rededicate them-selves to the DCCT and again achieve HbA_{1c} targets.

The Wheel that Squeaks Loudest

An additional realization has been the importance of attending not only to participants who are doing badly, but also to those who are doing well. Too often the assumption has been made that the latter require little help and that one should devote the majority of one's energy and time to difficult patients. The erroneousness of this tactic has been made clear by deteriorations in adherence alluded to earlier. Not all successful patients require close scrutiny, but most appreciate inquiries into their well-being. Conversely, patients who are doing poorly in the trial may absorb all efforts by clinic staff without improving substantially.

Changes in Treatment

Patient "burnout" is caused in some cases by the tedium of a difficult regimen. This can be offset by periodic changes of technology, staff, and treatment strategies. For example, the introduction of new reflectance meters, blood glucose analysis software, and injection devices has improved patients' glucose control as well as their outlook. Similarly, a change in staff can bring with it fresh treatment perspectives. However, all modifications need to be minimally disruptive (Shillitoe, 1988). Many patients are fiercely loyal to particular staff members, routines, and equipment. The potential benefits of changing treatment must be weighed against the emotional upheaval that may result in such cases.

Clinic Cohesiveness

It has become increasingly apparent that most participants work hardest when presented with a unified treatment plan. For example, patients who receive one message from the physician and contradictory or unnecessarily redundant information from the psychologist are more likely to be dissatisfied or confused. Clinic cohesiveness requires considerable time and effort. Staff members must meet as a group before, and sometimes after, individually seeing participants so that a plan can be fashioned, individual roles delegated amongst the staff, and patient reactions discussed.

The Role of Mental Health Professionals

The DCCT experience has underscored the wisdom of incorporating mental health professionals throughout the planning and the implementation of large-scale treatment studies. Their time commitment has been increased over the course of the trial, reflecting the many duties they have performed: (a) selection of endpoint measures to monitor adverse psychological effects (b) assistance with screening of study applicants (b) neurobehavioral testing (c) provision of individual and group counselling for patients (d) assistance with adherence-enhancing techniques (e) development of workshops to facilitate staff counselling skills and (g) maintenance of staff morale and effectiveness. Clearly, these individuals have served not only as participating team members but also as consultants, both at the clinic and national level. The DCCT experience has driven home the realization that each staff member must act, periodically, as a psychologist, psychiatrist, and social worker. This makes it all the more pressing that individuals who are specifically trained in these areas be available to guide their colleagues.

Summary and Conclusions

The DCCT provides an example of the myriad psychological issues endemic to long-term clinical trials. We attempted to select applicants carefully and educate them during screening. We considered it vital to monitor participant adherence, satisfaction, and well-being. As the trial has unfolded, both staff and patients have come to appreciate the challenges and dynamic nature of provider-patient relationships and adherence.

Readers who have participated in long-term clinical trials undoubtedly will recognize many of the issues enumerated above, and some will possess additional insights that are missing in this account. At the DCCT's inception, we searched the available psychological literature and found little that sprang from trial experience. Rather, most articles were based on theory or experiments. It is hoped that the lessons we and others have learned do not continue to require re-discovery with every new large-scale trial.

References

Bandura, A. (1989). Human agency in social cognitive theory. *American Psychologist*, **44**, 1175–1184.

Becker, M.H., & Janz, N.K. (1985). The health belief model applied to understanding diabetes regimen compliance. *The Diabetes Educator*, **11**, 41–47.

Bergner, M., Bobbitt, R.A., Carter, W.B., & Gilson, B.S. (1981). The Sickness Impact Profile: Development and final revision of a health status measure. *Medical Care*, **19**, 787–805.

Bradley, C. (1988). Stress and diabetes. In S. Fisher & J. Reason (Ed.), *Handbook of Life Stress, Cognition and Health* (Ch. 21; pp. 383–401). London: Wiley.

Brownlee-Duffeck, M., Peterson, L., Simonds, J.F., Goldstein, D., Kilo, C., & Hoette, S. (1987). The role of health beliefs in the regimen adherence and metabolic control of adolescents and adults with diabetes mellitus. *Journal of Consulting and Clinical Psychology*, **55**, 139–144.

The DCCT Research Group (1986). The Diabetes Control and Complications Trial (DCCT): Design and methodologic considerations for the feasibility phase. *Diabetes*, **35**, 530–545.

The DCCT Research Group (1987). The Diabetes Control and Complications Trial (DCCT): Results of the feasibility study. *Diabetes Care*, **10**, 1–19.

The DCCT Research Group (1988a): *DCCT Protocol*. Springfield, VA, U.S. Department of Commerce, National Technical Information Service, Accession No. PB 88–116462/AS.

The DCCT Research Group (1988b). Are continuing studies of metabolic control and microvascular complications in insulin-dependent diabetes mellitus justified?: The Diabetes Control and Complications Trial (DCCT). *New England Journal of Medicine*, **318**, 246–250.

The DCCT Research Group (1988c). Reliability and validity of a diabetes quality-of-life measure for the Diabetes Control and Complications Trial (DCCT). *Diabetes Care*, **11**, 725–732.

The DCCT Research Group (1988d). Weight gain associated with intensive therapy in the Diabetes Control and Complications Trial. *Diabetes Care*, **11**, 567–573.

The DCCT Research Group (1989). Implementation of a multi-component process to obtain informed consent in the Diabetes Control and Complications Trial. *Controlled Clinical Trials*, **10**, 83–96.

The DCCT Research Group (1990). Diabetes Control and Complications Trial (DCCT): Update. *Diabetes Care*, **13**, 427–433.

Derogatis, L.R., Rickels, K., & Rock, A. (1977). *The SCL-90-R: Administration, Scoring, and Procedures Manual I*. Baltimore: Clinical Psychosomatic Research.

Derogatis, L.R., Yevzeroff, H., & Wittelsberger, B. (1975). Social class, psychological disorder, and the nature of the psychopathologic indicator. *Journal of Consulting and Clinical Psychology*, **43**, 183–191.

DiMatteo, M.R., & DiNicola, D.D. (1982). *Achieving Patient Compliance: The Psychology of the Medical Practitioner's Role*. New York: Pergamon Press.

Eeg-Olofsson, O. (1977). Hypoglycemia and neurological disturbances in children with diabetes mellitus. *Acta Paediatrica Scandinavica* (Suppl. 270), 91–96.

Hauser, S.T., Jacobson, A.M., Lavori, P., Wolfsdorf, J., Herskowitz, R., Milley, J., et al. (1990). Adherence among children and adolescents with insulin-dependent diabetes mellitus over a four year longitudinal follow-up: II. Immediate and long-term linkages with the family milieu. *Journal of Pediatric Psychology*, **15**, 527–542.

Jacobson, A.M. (1986). Current status of psychosocial research in diabetes. *Diabetes Care*, **9**, 546–548.

Lorenz, R., & Siebert, C., Cleary, P., Santiago, J., & Heyse, S. for the DCCT Research Group (1988). Epidemiology of severe hypoglycemia in the DCCT. *Diabetes* **37** (Suppl. 1): **Abstract No. 3A**.

Mazze, R.S., Pasmantier, R., Murphy, J.A., & Shamoon, H. (1985). Self-monitoring of capillary blood glucose: Changing the performance of individuals with diabetes. *Diabetes Care*, **8**, 207–213.

Meichembaum, D., & Turk, D.C. (1987). *Facilitating Treatment Adherence: A Practitioner's Guidebook*. New York: Plenum Press.

Orme, C.M., & Binik, Y.M. (1989). Consistency of adherence across regimen demands. *Health Psychology*, **8**, 27–43.

Ryan, C.M. (1988). Neurobehavioral complications of Type I diabetes: Examination of possible risk factors. *Diabetes Care*, **11**, 86–93.

Ryan, C.M. (1990). Neuropsychological consequences and correlates of diabetes in childhood. In C.S. Holmes (Ed.), *Neuropsychological and Behavioral Aspects of Diabetes* (Ch 4, pp. 58–84). New York: Springer-Verlag.

Ryan, C.M., Adams, K.M., Heaton, R.K., Grant, I., Jacobson, A.M., and the DCCT Research Group (in press). Neurobehavioral assessment of medical patients in clinical trials: The DCCT experience. *Medical Trials*.

Schlenk, E.A., & Hart, L.K. (1984). Relationship between health locus of control, health value, and social support and compliance of persons with diabetes mellitus. *Diabetes Care*, **7**, 566–574.

Shillitoe, R.W. (1988). *Psychology and Diabetes: Psychosocial Factors in Management and Control*. London: Chapman and Hall.

Webb, K.L., Dobson, A.J., O'Connell, D.L., Tupling, H.E., Harris, G.W., Moxon, J.A., *et al.* (1984). Dietary compliance among insulin-dependent diabetics. *Journal of Chronic Diseases*, **37**, 633–643.

4

APPROPRIATE USE OF NEW TECHNOLOGIES

In the first of the next section's chapters, Chris Brewin, Clare Bradley and Philip Home offers a framework for systematic assessment of the needs of individuals with diabetes, to ensure that an available treatment is offered to a patient who needs it, but is not offered to one with no need of that treatment. A conceptual and methodological framework for needs assessment has recently been developed by Brewin and his colleagues at the Institute of Psychiatry, for assessment of needs of people with psychiatric disorders. Here, in collaboration with a psychologist having a special interest in diabetes (Bradley) and a diabetologist (Home), this framework is adapted to the issues of diabetes management. The diabetes needs' assessment framework offered here awaits evaluation of its use in a diabetes clinic, to determine its usefulness as a tool for promoting optimal care of people with diabetes by encouraging appropriate (and discouraging inappropriate) use of available treatments.

The following chapter by Theresa Marteau considers the costs as well as the benefits that can be associated with the use of new technologies. Development of a new technology is only the first step on the path towards effective use of the technology. Drawing on the literature concerned with technology in other fields of medicine as well as in diabetes care, Marteau highlights the importance of considering patient and staff attitudes to new technologies and the need for awareness of the possible barriers and adverse consequences associated with new technologies, if appropriate implementation of new technological developments is to be facilitated to the best advantage of all concerned.

The third chapter by Kirsten Staehr Johansen of the World Health Organisation takes a more global view of the need to maximise appropriate use of techology in health care services. The WHO definition of appropriate technology includes the appropriateness of the technology to a particular country's needs and resources. The targets and recommendations of the WHO emphasize the importance of technology assessment in multinational studies; this includes not only evaluation of the effects of the technology on metabolic control and other clinical criteria but also on economic and psychosocial variables, including indices of 'quality of life'. One of the few studies which has included measures of all these variables, a multicentre European randomised cross-over study comparing the effects of treatment with continuous subcutaneous insulin infusion pumps with that of conventional injection treatment, is described and offered as a model for appropriate technology assessment both within diabetes care and, more generally in research evaluating the appropriate use of technology in other health services.

Measuring Needs in Patients with Diabetes

Chris R. Brewin, Clare Bradley, and Philip D. Home
MRC Social and Community Psychiatry Unit, Institute of Psychiatry, London: Joint appointment between Department of General Practice, UMDS, Guy's Campus, and Department of Psychology, Royal Holloway and Bedford New College; University of London: Department of Medicine, University of Newcastle upon Tyne, UK.

Providers of services are increasingly being enjoined to measure the effectiveness and the efficiency with which they are meeting their patients' needs. But to date there has been little discussion of what is meant by a need and how to go about measuring them. In this chapter we shall first discuss the concept of need and then describe how an instrument designed for measuring the needs of the long-term mentally ill could be adapted to assess the needs of patients with diabetes.

Dictionary definitions of 'need' indicate that the term has a range of connotations, including a state of want or destitution, a condition requiring some extraneous aid, and an imperative call or demand for some provision. In ordinary language, therefore, the term is ambiguous about the extent to which action is required.

Discussions of need as applied to health have identified other important distinctions, such as that between patient-assessed and provider-assessed need. In a well-known article Bradshaw (1972) has further distinguished two sorts of patient-assessed need, 'felt' need and 'expressed' need. The former is only experienced, whereas the latter is both experienced and communicated. Bradshaw also identifies two kinds of externally-defined need, 'normative' (based on the judgement of professionals such as psychiatrists) and 'comparative' (based on comparison with other individuals or reference groups). As Mägi and Allander (1981) point out, need statements imply both factual and value elements. That is to say, need statements may describe an actual state of affairs but they also depend on an implicit or explicit value system which determines which states of affairs are considered acceptable and which courses of action are considered appropriate. Need, then, according to this approach, can never be objectively defined but must be understood in terms of the person or group making the judgement.

Other health economists (e.g. Matthew, 1971) have suggested that need should be distinguished from 'demand' on the one hand and 'service utilisation' on the other. Patients may demand treatments that in the judgement of clinicians they do not need, and service utilisation may either underestimate or overestimate actual need, depending on such factors as resource availability, acceptability of treatment, physician and patient education, etc. In this view needs should be normatively defined by clinicians, and should depend on the existence of effective and acceptable treatments. Thus a patient with terminal, inoperable cancer would not be judged to have a need for treatment although they might be judged to have a need for pain relief, counselling, or other interventions aimed at related problems.

The MRC Needs Assessment Procedure

One current approach to measuring need in long-term psychiatric patients has been developed from the earlier work of John Wing on the planning and evaluation of psychiatric services (Wing, 1972, 1978, 1986). The present model involves a four-stage process. At the first stage investigators identify the presence of 'social disablement', defined as lowered physical, psychological, and social functioning, compared with what would ordinarily be expected, in a particular society, of a typical individual. The second stage is concerned with the identification of methods of 'care' that are thought to be effective and acceptable means of reducing or containing the components of social disablement. The term 'care' is used in a broad sense to encompass all interventions from the most active treatment to the most passive form of shelter. At the third stage the therapeutic agents (e.g. psychiatrists, general practitioners, nurses etc.) capable of undertaking these interventions are identified. Finally, the appropriate organisation of agents into agencies (e.g. self-help groups, day hospitals, hostels) for the coordinated delivery of care is considered. These agencies collectively form the total 'need for service' of the individual patient. In this chapter we will outline the procedures developed for assessing needs for items of care. A fuller description and rationale can be found in Brewin *et al.* (1987) and an account of the Camberwell High Contact Survey, using the data generated by these procedures, in Brewin *et al.* (1988).

Social disablement may be considered as a series of 'wants' or 'problems' presented by the individual patient. In some cases these are accompanied by the 'wants' and 'problems' of relatives who live with or take care of the patient. These wants and problems are then legitimised as 'needs' for care and services by others – in this case by professionals who are afforded allocative discretionary powers through the exercise of their expertise. In many circumstances – particularly in non-technical areas – the individual's articulation of wants corresponds totally with the judgments of professionals concerning needs. Nonetheless, in our model, the individual cannot be the final arbiter of needs, for their resolution depends on (a) expert knowledge, (b) the integration of information from patients, families, and involved professionals, and (c) the reconciliation of competing wants. Our procedure, then, relies on professional judgment – Bradshaw's 'normative' need – and makes the assumption that a substantial clinical consensus among 'experts' is achievable. It is an attempt to formalise and structure what is good clinical practice.

Our first task was therefore to generate basic rules of good practice. In the care of the long-term mentally ill it is rarely the case that there exist treatments of scientifically proven efficacy, and care is usually provided in a context of multiple clinical, social and economic problems. These considerations led to a model of ideal clinical practice in the care of the long-term mentally ill. Its purpose was to identify a small number of basic principles in the care and treatment of common symptoms, behaviour problems, and behaviour deficits. We did not claim that our model was capable of encompassing all eventualities or crises that might arise, nor that it would remove the necessity for staff to respond flexibly and imaginatively to each individual.

The model had three elements. First, the patient's clinical and social functioning should be regularly and systematically assessed in order to identify areas of improvement or deterioration. General goals consisted of the amelioration of symptoms and distress, and the development of self-care, social, and occupational skills. Patients' own perceptions of their problems and their priorities for action should feature prominently, however, so that treatment plans would be based on the goals of both patients and staff. Second, an identified deficit or problem should prompt a list of potential interventions, ranging from active therapy or training to the provision of support and shelter. The failure or only partial success of one intervention should lead automatically, after a specified period of time, to trials of other interventions from the list. Third, failure or only partial success of all appropriate forms of care should trigger future intervention at regular intervals in the hope that the patient would be more able to utilize help or that the help offered would be more in accord with the patient's own priorities.

Measuring Needs for Care

Our definition of need is based on the principle that, for need to exist, some item of care must be identified that might reduce or ameliorate social disablement. In other words, actions by care staff are not legitimised simply by the existence of social disablement, but by a further set of rules indicating whether action is appropriate or inappropriate. This leads to the following definitions of need for care:

1. Need is present when (a) a patient's functioning (social disablement) falls below or threatens to fall below some minimum specified level, and (b) this is due to a remediable, or potentially remediable, cause.
2. A need (as defined above) is met when it has attracted some at least partly effective item of care, and when no other items of care of greater potential effectiveness exist.

3. A need (as defined above) is unmet when it has attracted only partly effective or no item of care and when other items of care of greater potential effectiveness exist.

Figure 1 *Assessment of Functioning, Assessment of Interventions, and Need Status*

Assessment of functioning	Assessment of interventions	Need status
No problem or mild problem	None employed	No need
Significant current or recent problem	None even partly effective	No meetable need
	Some potentially fully effective	Met need
	None fully effective: no alternatives	Met need
	None fully effective: alternatives available	Unmet need for treatment
Level of functioning not known		Unmet need for assessment

These definitions are represented in Figure 1, which specifies how assessments of social disablement and assessments of items of care are combined to yield judgements concerning need. Figure 1 implies the necessity for assumptions about which areas of social disablement are important, which interventions are appropriate for different types of social disablement, and what constitutes effectiveness.

Assessing Social Disablement

Behind the definition of this concept lie notions of physical and psychological health, and of a 'core of competence'. For our purposes, these notions were conceived as minimal acceptable levels of health and competence. Thus, health was defined in terms of the absence of various kinds of symptoms rather than in terms of the achievement of positive health goals. Similarly, the core of competence was defined in terms of the minimum skills required to function independently in the community, rather than in terms of higher level skills that might maximise the individual's autonomy and quality of life. Ratings, based on standardised psychiatric assessments carried out with patients and key informants, reflected whether symptoms were current (i.e. were present in the past month), absent in the past month but recently present, or completely absent. The distinction between 'current' and 'recent' symptoms is necessary in order that items of care offered for purely preventive purposes can be rated appropriately.

Assessing Items of Care

In each area of social disablement the Needs for Care assessment specifies a list of 2–8 appropriate items of care, covering such diverse types of care as medication, counselling, behaviour programmes, remedial education, and the provision of a sheltered environment. Our aim was to be over- rather than under-inclusive, and this meant including items of care not necessarily in widespread use, although we judged them to be generally acceptable to professionals.

Figure 2   *Ratings Given to Individual Items of Care*

---

0 =   Not appropriate and not provided
1 =   Currently being provided and effective or potentially effective
2 =   Currently being provided but has proved to be insufficient by itself after 3 months trial
3 =   Offered during past year but unacceptable to patient
4 =   Given adequate trial in past 2 years and proved ineffective.
5 =   Provided inappropriately and not worth continuing
6 =   Appropriate now but not given adequate or recent trial

Each item of care receives a single rating (see Figure 2) by the investigator that indicates whether or not it has been tried, how effective it was, whether or not it was acceptable to the patient, and whether or not it is currently appropriate. This rating is based on an interview with a key worker or with other appropriate staff. The investigator must determine whether items of care have received an adequate trial from a properly qualified or supervised person, and must solicit evidence for the effectiveness or otherwise of the intervention. Rules exist to help decide how long to persevere with one form of care before trying another, and to decide when ineffective or unacceptable items of care should be tried or offered again. Staff members are similarly questioned about the appropriateness of the various alternative items of care, but the final judgement on the rating is the investigator's.

Assessing Need Status

Need status in each area of social disablement is derived algorithmically from consideration of the level of disablement and the ratings given to items of care. Effectively, the level of disablement is matched with the level of care provided, permitting an estimate of under-, over-, or appropriate provision. Primary need status falls into 4 categories, 'met need', 'unmet need', 'no need', and 'no meetable need' (the last two categories have in previous reports been collapsed together as 'no need'). 'Met need' indicates that there is current or recent disablement, but that the patient is receiving a fully effective or potentially fully effective item of care. When the items of care being employed are clearly insufficient, although continuing input is required, a rating of 'met need' indicates that no other items of care of greater potential effectiveness exist. 'Unmet need' indicates that there is current disablement, that no current items of care are fully effective (although they may well be worth continuing), and that potentially more effective alternatives do exist. An 'unmet need' for assessment is also rated when the presence or absence of current disablement is not known. Finally, 'no need' indicates that there is no disablement, and 'no meetable need' that there is disablement but that there are no items of care which are currently at all feasible and appropriate.

The fact that wants or problems can only be legitimised as needs if there are currently feasible and appropriate interventions deserves further comment. This principle follows logically from our definition of need as a requirement for some specifiable form of care. Hence, if all forms of care are inappropriate, have proven to be completely ineffective, or have been refused by the patient, need cannot be said to exist. Instead, the individual will be rated by our methods as having a problem but no meetable need. An example from another area of medicine will illustrate this situation. Patients with terminal cancers may *want* a cure, but from the perspective of the service providers they do not have a meetable *need* for a cure so long as the cancer is untreatable by currently available methods. The same patients may, on the other hand, be in pain and distressed, two problems for which interventions do exist. It therefore makes sense to say that they have a need for pain relief and for counselling. To say that terminal cancer patients *need* a cure may be a useful statement for clinical researchers who can set about inventing or developing one. The statement has little meaning for clinicians or planners, however, since there are no immediate service implications other than a possible requirement for psychosocial support.

Problems with no associated meetable needs do occur from time to time with the long-term mentally ill (Brewin *et al.*, 1988). While recognising the limitations of current forms of care, this in no way vitiates the obligation of agents to develop new and more effective interventions, or to persevere in the future with interventions that may have been unacceptable or ineffective in the past. Indeed, future repetitions of the Needs for Care Assessment would make this duty explicit. The concept of a problem with no meetable need highlights the important fact that, at least in the care of the long-term mentally ill, professional knowledge and practice are inadequate to meet all our patients' problems.

In addition to the primary need status, the assessment permits three secondary judgements to be made in each area of disablement. Of these the most important is *overprovision* which is rated whenever one or more items of care are judged as being superfluous. In some cases this will be because an item of care continues to be given even though it is not targeted at a specific problem or appears to be completely ineffective. In other cases the rating reflects that the patient is in receipt of an item of care even though there has been no disablement for a considerable period of time, and there is no apparent danger of relapse. In the Camberwell High Contact Study (Brewin *et al.*, 1988) instances of overprovision, mainly for medication, were found to be as common as were unmet needs for treatment.

Reliability and Validity

Initial data on the reliability and validity of the assessment are presented in Brewin *et al.* (1987, 1988). Clearly, estimates of validity can only be limited ones given that by definition need involves the making of value judgements and that no other comparable definitions and measures of need exist. Some recent data do, however, shed light on the reliability of the procedure. Lesage *et al.* (in press) employed an Italian version of the assessment in a study of psychiatric services in South Verona. The primary need status of sixty-one identified problems found in 20 patients was independently rated by one Camberwell-trained judge and by two Italian judges. The three judges showed a high level of agreement (kappa = .92, p<.0001), reliably identifying a relatively high level of unmet need among this subset of problems.

The needs of patients from the same area but living on different sides of an administrative boundary and attending the same day hospital have recently been assessed in two independent studies. One group (N=11) were assessed as part of the Camberwell High Contact Study (Brewin *et al.*, 1988; Brugha *et al.*, 1988) and the other (N=66) as part of a survey of day care in an inner city (Wainwright, Holloway, and Brugha, 1988). In both studies the MRC Needs for Care Assessment produced similar mean numbers of problems per patient with similar percentages of unmet needs, suggesting that, when used by suitably trained investigators, the measure is reliable and is robust enough to tolerate minor procedural deviations.

Measuring Needs for Care in Diabetes

Caring for individuals with diabetes mellitus shares a number of character-istics with caring for the long-term mentally ill. In both cases the typical patient will have a long history of illness, during which time he or she will have made a series of unique decisions and adjustments in the attempt to live with the illness. Recent research emphasizes the importance of the coping strategies adopted by the mentally ill patient to control his or her symptoms – although the degree of patient self-management is rarely as great as in diabetes, similar processes appear to be operative. In both cases the goals of patients and care staff will not always coincide, and optimum care will often involve considerable negotiation to settle on the alternatives that make the best compromise between the concerns of the clinician and the concerns of the patient. Thus our strategy of making repeated regular assessments, specifying a range of possible interventions for each of a number of problems, and requiring clinicians exhaustively to consider each intervention whenever clinical targets are not being met, appears to be applicable in principle to diabetes care. Instead of the 20 areas of functioning covered in the original assessment, however, we believe that the routine practice of diabetologists could be covered in 6 areas, each with an associated list of appropriate interventions: a) metabolic control, b) foot care, c) eye care, d) cardiac function, e) renal function, and f) sexual problems. Other associated and coincident illness could be dealt with as additional needs.

Figure 3   *Suggested Interventions for Problems with Unacceptable Metabolic Control of Diabetes*

Education about reasons for and means of achieving control
Systematic dietary counselling
Exercise programme
Weight reduction support group
Change amount of insulin/change number of tablets/change to insulin from
        tablets
Change type of insulin/change type of tablets/start tablets
Systematic blood glucose monitoring
Change injection regimen
Pen injector
Social counselling
Referral to psychologist for stress, weight, etc.
Standard insulin pump
Programmable pump
Other

Assessing at regular intervals the level of functioning (no problem, recent problem, or current problem) in each area could be achieved using standard diagnostic tests with commonly agreed thresholds to denote the presence of a problem. For example, it might be agreed that a problem in the area of metabolic control would be rated whenever there had been recent hypoglycaemic episodes *or* haemoglobin A_1 exceeding the European standard of 8.5% (Alberti and Gries, 1988), which would indicate unacceptably high average blood glucose levels over the past 6 to 8 weeks. Presence of a problem would trigger consideration of a list of interventions, for example those in Figure 3.

Each intervention would then be given one of the ratings presented in Figure 2, indicating whether it had received an adequate and recent trial, whether it was acceptable to the patient, whether it was partially effective and worth continuing or ineffective and not worth continuing, or whether it was clinically inappropriate (for example, several of the interventions aimed at achieving better metabolic control would be inappropriate for patients with Type 2 diabetes). These ratings would then be combined to generate judgements of unmet need, met need, or no need. Overprovision could also be rated if desired.

A similar procedure would then be followed for the other areas of functioning, where different kinds of intervention would be appropriate. Suggestions for these interventions are given in Figure 4. The resulting output would be in the form of 6 need status judgements per patient, together with an indication of any interventions that had not received adequate trial despite unmet need or that were overprovided.

This procedure allows for the fact that clinicians may want to continue with a variety of interventions, none of which may be fully effective, in addition to testing the effects of additional interventions. Rating a patient as having an unmet need does not imply that existing interventions are superfluous, merely that they are insufficient. In practice there may be difficulties in assessing effectiveness because certain interventions are provided at the same time in the form of a standard package. Although this approach has its merits, introducing several interventions concurrently places heavy demands on patients' ability to remember and comprehend the information they have been given, a situation that has been shown to reduce adherence. We suggest that, where clinically justified, attempts should be made to introduce and assess interventions serially rather than in parallel. Thus, an educational intervention would be followed by knowledge tests as well as clinical assessments; if it were then shown that the patient's knowledge was adequate but that metabolic control was still poor, education would cease and another intervention such as systematic dietary counselling could be attempted, to be followed by detailed monitoring of patients' actual diet during a typical week. If such an approach is not followed, it may be difficult to distinguish between effective and ineffective parts of the total therapeutic package, with a consequent over-burdening of the patient and a waste of limited resources.

Perhaps the best way of illustrating the operation of the needs for care assessment is to consider the case of a hypothetical patient Mr S. Mr S has a history of poor control and at his next clinic visit his HbA_1 is 13.0%, which according to our agreed threshold constitutes a current problem in metabolic control. Interventions that have been tried in the past 2 years and found to be

Figure 4   *Suggested Interventions for Other Areas of Functioning**

Foot care

Education on foot care	Chiropody
Supervised examination of feet	Referral to vascular
Skin/ulcer care	surgeon
Shoe choice	Deformity correction
Other	Amputation

Eye care

Referral to ophthalmologist	Visual aids
Other	

Cardiac function

Risk factor control/education	Hypertension control
Stress management	Angina management
Smoking cessation group	Heart failure management
Other	Referral to cardiologist

Renal function

Dietary control (protein)	Hypertension control
Other infection control	Nephrological referral

Sexual problems

Psychosexual counselling	Erection aids
Self-injection with papaverine	Surgical intervention
Other	

* It is assumed that metabolic control is receiving attention as a separate area of functioning (see Figure 3)

ineffective (rating 4) are education concerning the reasons for achieving control and changes in the amount and type of insulin. One year ago Mr S agreed to changes in the injection regimen coupled with systematic blood glucose monitoring, which have proved to be partially but not fully effective in reducing blood glucose levels and are worth continuing (rating 2). Stress counselling does not appear to be appropriate (rating 0) since there are no reported problems that are currently causing trouble. The following interventions appear to be appropriate but have not received an adequate or recent trial (rating 7): systematic dietary counselling, pen injectors, and standard or programmable pumps. On questioning, Mr S, who lives alone, appears to have a very unsophisticated notion about diet and menu planning, and you suspect that considerable improvement might follow from a more appropriate balancing of carbohydrate diet and insulin dose. He is open to this suggestion, and both you and he agree that systematic dietary counselling might be the most helpful step at this stage.

On routine clinical examination there is no problem or need in the areas of foot care or cardiac function. There are, however, clear signs of progressive retinopathy that have not been apparent before, indicating a current problem in this area and an unmet need for referral to an ophthalmologist. You review Mr S's kidney function and find evidence of microalbuminuria. His blood pressure control is excellent and requires no intervention but his high protein intake suggests a need for some modification. This is also therefore rated as an unmet need. A few months ago Mr S reported sexual difficulties and you have arranged for him to have psychosexual counselling. It is too early to say whether this will be effective and it is therefore rated as potentially effective (rating 1), so that the need is met.

We summarise the results of the needs assessment in Figure 5. This indicates that Mr. S has four problems, of which one is a met need and three are unmet needs. Such a chart could be completed at each clinic visit, providing a record of the care plan followed and the results of each intervention undertaken. It should be noted that in our procedure unmet needs are simply *recommendations for action*, and it will not be known until follow-up assessments are completed whether the new intervention has been effective in meeting the need, whether the need remains unmet, or whether it is unmeetable.

Figure 5   *Summary of the Problem and Need Status of Mr S.*

Area of functioning	Problem status	Need status	Intervention
Metabolic control	Current problem	Unmet need	Dietary counselling
Foot care	No problem	No need	
Eye care	Current problem	Unmet need	Referral to ophthalmologist
Cardiac function	No problem	No need	
Renal function	Current problem	Unmet need	Dietary change
Sexual problems	Current problem	Met need	Psycho-sexual counselling

Discussion

What systematic needs assessment has to offer is an explicit care plan against which can be measured the actions of a clinical team. Alternatively it can be used to compare the actions of different clinical teams, or different hospitals. We would not wish to claim, any more than in the case of the long-term mentally ill, that the scheme we have outlined for diabetes is adequate to meet all clinical situations, or that it represents the best possible standard of care. Rather, we see it as attempting to establish a baseline below which levels of care should not fall. It is a way of monitoring whether basic standards are being maintained, and identifying particular forms of care for which there may be a particular need within a hospital or health district.

The monitoring of needs is a sensitive exercise: scanning too wide or too often can lead to an inappropriate action on ephemeral or 'low priority' problems that might remit spontaneously. Equally, failing to monitor needs sufficiently regularly can lead to misuse of limited resources, and to the danger that patients' autonomy will be reduced rather than enhanced. The Royal College of Psychiatrists recently expressed concern about these issues in a report on deinstitutionalisation policies now gaining pace in Britain, where it drew attention to the 'fine line between liberty and neglect'. Further research is required to determine whether the MRC procedures strike the right balance between identifying too few and too many needs.

Among the limitations of our procedures is that, in order to be useful clinically, they must be repeated at regular intervals. Needs for care in particular are not static but are expected to change in response to improvement and deterioration in clinical condition, to significant changes in patients' lives, and to many other factors. This suggests that for clinical purposes needs for care assessments should be repeated at six-monthly or yearly intervals. This would almost certainly be true of other similar assessments, however.

A second limitation is that relatively little attention appears to be paid to patients' own definitions of their 'needs' – indeed, these would be labelled as 'wants' rather than as needs in our terminology. We have explained that one reason for our preference for 'expert-defined' need is because service providers allocate limited resources and have to decide what is clinically feasible. We also believe it essential that services should start out with a clear idea of potential areas of need rather than solely relying on patients to articulate them. While some patients would be more than able to articulate their wants, it is unrealistic to expect all to do so regardless of such factors as their education, clinical condition, and expectations. We have therefore opted for a procedure that in almost all cases can use information supplied by the patient to identify potential problem areas, and recognises patients' rights to veto suggested interventions. There is also scope for patients' unique problems, whether raised by themselves or by members of staff, to be included as additional needs.

From an organisational and clinical perspective, the monitoring of needs is an iterative process by which alternative solutions to eradicate patients' problems, and ways of coordinating and effectively implementing the appropriate interventions, are assessed. Despite the limitations inevitable in such a recently developed procedure, we are hopeful that the MRC Needs for Care Assessment does have the potential to improve general standards of care and could enable services to be evaluated and compared in a meaningful way.

Summary and Conclusions

Needs assessments are a logical next step from assessing blood glucose levels and other clinical and laboratory data. Rather than simply measuring how the patient is functioning, they also record clinical actions taken and hence can provide information on how adequately a clinical team has responded to a set of problems. In each of several areas of functioning (e.g., metabolic control, complications), patients can be rated as having:

1. No need (functioning is within acceptable limits).
2. Met need (a problem is being treated with a potentially fully effective item of care, or is being treated with a partially effective item of care and no other interventions of greater potential effectiveness exist).
3. Unmet need (a problem is being treated with an ineffective or only partially effective item of care, and other interventions of greater potential effectiveness exist).

We have described the development of a comprehensive needs assessment instrument for patients with other chronic problems (the long-term mentally ill) and outline how the same approach could be applied to diabetes care.

References

Alberti, K.G.M.M. and Gries, F.A. (1988). Management of non-insulin dependent diabetes in Europe: A consensus view. *Diabetic Medicine*, 5 275–281.

Bradshaw, J. (1972). A taxonomy of social need. In G. McLachlan (ed.), *Problems and progress in medical care* (Volume 7). London: Oxford University Press.

Brewin, C.R., Wing, J.K., Mangen, S.P., Brugha, T.S. and MacCarthy, B. (1987). Principles and practice of measuring needs in the long-term mentally ill: The MRC Needs for Care Assessment. *Psychological Medicine*, 17 971–981.

Brewin, C.R., Wing, J.K., Mangen, S.P., Brugha, T.S., MacCarthy, B. and Lesage, A. (1988). Needs for care among the long-term mentally ill: A report from the Camberwell High Contact Survey. *Psychological Medicine* 18, 457–468.

Lesage, A., Mignolli, G., Faccincani, C. and Tansella, M. (in press). Standardised assessment of the needs for care in a cohort of patients with schizophrenic psychoses. *Psychological Medicine*.

Mägi, M. and Allander, E. (1981). Towards a theory of perceived and medically defined need. *Sociology of Health and Illness*, 3 49–71.

Matthew, G.K. (1971). Measuring need and evaluating services. In G. McLachlan (ed.), *Portfolio for health*. London: O.U.P.

Wainwright, T., Holloway, F. and Brugha, T.S. (1988). Day care in an inner city. In A. Lavender and F. Holloway (eds.), *Community Care in Practice: Services for the continuing care client*. Chichester: Wiley.

Wing, J.K. (1972). Principles of evaluation. In J.K. Wing and A.M. Hailey (eds.), *Evaluating a Community Psychiatric Service*. Oxford: Oxford University Press.

Wing, J.K. (1978). Medical and social science and medical and social care. In J. Barnes and N. Connelly (eds.), *Social Care Research*. London: Bedford Square Press.

Wing, J.K. (1986). The cycle of planning and evaluation. In G. Wilkinson and H. Freeman (eds.), *The Provision of Mental Health Services in Britain: The Way Ahead*. London: Gaskell.

The Double-Edged Sword
of Technology in Health Care

Theresa M. Marteau

Health Psychology Unit, Royal Free Hospital School of Medicine, London NW3 2QG, UK.

For, medicine being a compendium of the successive and contradictory mistakes of medical practitioners, when we summon the wisest of them to our aid, the chances are that we may be relying on a scientific truth the error of which will be recognised in a few years' time. So that to believe in medicine would be the height of folly, if not to believe in it were not greater folly still, for from this mass of errors there have emerged in the course of time many truths.

Proust, The Guermenates Way I

The benefits that technology has brought to medical care are widely acclaimed and provide the impetus to continuing investment in research and developments. This is as evident in relation to diabetes as to other areas of care. But new technologies bring in their wake new issues for health professionals as well as patients. Evaluation of new technologies has been unsystematic; and where they have been evaluated, the focus has tended to be narrow, largely neglecting psychological and social factors (Council for Science and Society, 1982). Taking the example of screening, the outcomes will include participants' emotional and behavioural responses as well as morbidity and mortality figures, all of which need to be included in any assessment of the benefits and costs of screening (Marteau, 1989). The relative neglect of psychological factors in the breast and cervical screening programmes is, in part, responsible for the poor uptake and, in turn, relative inaffectiveness of these programmes (Fallowfield, 1988; Johnston, 1989). Consideration of psychological factors is therefore an essential part of evaluating any technology, as well as planning its successful implementation.

This chapter will explore some of the issues raised by technology for patients and health professionals, using examples from diabetes as well as other areas of health care.

The Decision to use a New Technology

In the development stages of a new technology, there may be limited information about its effectiveness and the risks entailed in its use. In addition, a new
technology such as the continuous subcutaneous insulin infusion pump
involves active patient participation. For reasons such as these, patients need
to be as fully informed as possible to make a decision about whether and when
to use a new technology. There are however several factors that militate
against this, namely the enthusiasm of many patients for medical technology,
doctors' enthusiasm for new technology, and the traditional roles of active
doctor and passive patient.

There is invariably pressure to apply new technology, even without full
evaluation, when it holds out some prospect of benefit. This 'tendency to take
action, whatever the costs if it offers even a slight possibility of utility' has
been labelled the technological imperative (Mechanic, 1979). Tymstra (1989)
suggests that people are motivated to follow virtually all diagnostic or therapeutic possibilities to avoid a feeling of regret, an important motivational factor
in the choices people make.

In addition to patients' enthusiasm, doctors' positive attitudes to new technology are likely to influence the way that they seek patients' consent to its
use. One of the factors influencing patients' treatment decisions is the way or
manner in which relevant risk information is provided (McNeil et al., 1982).
For example, given the same risks, if the possible outcome is expressed in
terms of likely success as opposed to likely failure, patients and doctors are
more likely to choose that option (Marteau, 1989a). Thus, doctors may unwittingly persuade patients just by the manner in which they present the facts
about a treatment.

Doctors are powerful figures for patients. This can make it difficult for
some patients to contradict or express a choice that they feel the doctor would
not make. In addition, patients frequently wish to please the doctor, perhaps to
repay help given, or in the hope that the doctor will continue to help them.

Regardless of the attitudes of patients and doctors towards new technologies, the role of doctors and patients is traditionally one that does not encourage
patients to have an active part in decision-making. Such a situation is likely to
be fostered by both doctors' and patients' expectations of appropriate behaviour. While training doctors in communication skills has attempted to teach
doctors to elicit patients' perspectives, the more dramatic changes in the
consultation have occurred following patient training. Several studies have
documented that following brief training, patients take a more active part in
consultations, in particular they ask more questions (Roter, 1977; Greenfield
et al., 1985). In one study, 73 patients with diabetes were randomly allocated
either to an experimental or a control group (Greenfield et al., 1988). The
experimental group received two 20 minute training sessions, designed to
motivate them to negotiate medical decisions, to be inquisitive and to assert
control in the doctor-patient relationship. Patients in the experimental group

elicited significantly more information from their doctors and subsequently reported fewer limitations on their lives from their disease. Three months later, their blood glucose control was significantly better than that of the control group.

There is some debate about the relative merits of involving patients in difficult decisions concerning their care. It has been argued, for example, that it is unethical to invite patients to participate in randomised controlled trials when they have been recently diagnosed with cancer, the decision of whether to participate and the implication that medical knowledge is far from perfect, serving to raise pre-existing anxieties (Baum *et al.,* 1989). There are however few empirical data to support this view (Marteau, 1989b). Some patients prefer not to make treatment choices, preferring to leave this to doctors.The size of this group is likely to depend upon the nature of the decision in question. In a study of the psychological effects of treatment choice in women with breast cancer, no adverse consequences of making a decision were found for these patients (Fallowfield *et al.,* 1990). In another study of women with breast cancer, psychological benefits were found in women who took explicit responsibility for their treatment decisions (Deadman-Spall *et al.,* 1990).

Perhaps the consequences for patients in their involvement in decisions will be influenced by the outcome: if it is positive, patients may benefit from having been involved in the initial decision, but if the outcome is negative, patients may feel in part to blame, having been involved in that decision. For some technologies, such as organ transplants and pump implants, the failure rate may be particularly high. Studies of the consequences of decisions that result in failure suggest that individuals protect themselves by the way they perceive the outcome or their part in it (Brehm, 1956; Festinger and Carlsmith, 1959). In medical contexts, a patient whose treatment fails may react in one of several ways in order to reduce its impact: (a) minimise their responsibility and blame the doctor; (b) minimise the decision, and decide that no decision was really made; or (c) decide that the consequences were not very severe. The few studies that have addressed this question suggest that there is no adverse consequence for patients when the outcome of their treatment choice is negative. In a retrospective study of 29 patients with kidney failure, those whose transplant failed recalled their initial decision as one where they had little choice in contrast with the recollections of patients whose transplants were successful (Wagener &Taylor, 1986). Similar findings are evident in studies of patients and their relatives following failed liver transplants (Tymstra, 1989). Research on hindsight biases shows that when people know the outcome of a situation, they exaggerate in retrospect what could have been anticipated (Fishchoff, 1982). This implies that in order for patients to be cognitively protected from adverse outcomes, they must understand all possible outcomes, thereby knowing in advance what negative consequences are possible.

A further argument for patients to be actively involved in these decisions is that staff and patients are likely to differ in their perceptions of the need for the technology and their goals of treatment. That patients and doctors may disagree on the need for an intervention was illustrated in a study concerning the appropriateness of facial plastic surgery for children with Down's syndrome (Pueschel *et al.*, 1986). While almost half the paediatricians were in favour of such a procedure, only 13% of parents were. In managing diabetes in their children, parents' goals of treatment differed from those of doctors, parents' goals reflecting an avoidance of hypoglycaemia, doctors' goals reflecting an avoidance of hyperglycaemia (Marteau *et al.*, 1987).

Effects of Technology on Patients

The acceptability of any technology, patients' responses to it, and its effectiveness, will vary according to both the technology and characteristics of the patient.

Whether a piece of equipment is noticeable will be one factor influencing responses to it. For example, for some patients, the externally worn CSII pumps were unacceptable, having the potential to draw attention to the fact that the individual has diabetes, an otherwise largely hidden disease. Given the tendency for people to hold negative attitudes towards those with a disease (Tringo, 1970), for some patients social attitudes will be the most important consideration in their use of technology that has the potential to reveal their condition.

Some technologies allow observation and measurement of parts of the body previously accessible only by invasive methods, such as the new scanning devices of ultrasound and magnetic resonance imaging. Patients rely heavily upon staff for interpretation of these data. Inherent in the use of such techniques is the possibility of holding secrets from patients, a potential that has been used in some studies in which patients have tested their blood glucose levels on devices that unbeknown to them have been recording the measurements made (Mazze, 1984). This has revealed a discrepancy between what patients have recorded as their results and their actual results, as objectively recorded. Interpretation of these findings have lead to the use of such terms as falsification and cheating. An alternative interpretation is that patients are presenting an optimistic view of their progress to both themselves and their carers and perhaps protecting all those involved from a sense of failure in the face of disappointing results. Such a cognitive bias is a well-described phenomenon that most people engage in (Weinstein, 1982), including health professionals, who for example view their skills with more confidence than is justified on objective assessment (Marteau *et al.*, 1989). Studies that involve the possibility of confronting patients with discrepancies in their own accounts of their progress hold the potential to undermine the trust upon which the doctor-patient relationship is based, without which all attempts to help may founder. Such studies allow technology to assume a role of aiding the doctor against the patient, rather than as an aid for both doctor and patient to use to achieve the patients' goals.

The intended purpose of some technology is to reveal the hidden, with the purpose of monitoring some event and accordingly exerting some control over it. This is a characteristic of several new technological developments in diabetes, including blood glucose measuring devices (from reagent strips to memory blood glucose meters) and glucose sensors. For some people this will enhance their sense of control; for others it may lead to a sense of anxiety, and helplessness, as well as a constant reminder of being different. Implantable blood glucose sensors with hypoglycaemia alarms may be welcomed by some patients. Observation of parents with children with apnea alarms suggests that, for some, such alarms keep anxiety levels raised by acting as a constant reminder to parents of their children's mortality. Information about the ability or perceived ability to act to improve the outcome may discourage some patients (Bandura, 1977). For those who feel unable to improve their blood glucose levels, measurement may underline feelings of failure. In discussing the results of their study of CSII in children and adolescents, Davis and colleagues (1984) suggested that "a thought should be spared for those children who could not tolerate the technique, because it is possible for them to consider themselves 'failures' and to become demoralised further." There is some evidence that those who have a high need for control over outcomes respond less favourably to diabetes (Lowry & Ducette, 1976).

Studies that have evaluated the use of computers in consultations for accessing and updating patient records have generally not found any adverse effects (Rethans et al., 1988; Brownbridge et al., 1985). However, two studies found that patients with less positive attitudes towards computers reported higher levels of stress after consultations in which doctors used computers compared with patients with more positive attitudes (Cruickshank, 1982; Brownbridge et al., 1985). The duration of consultations in which the doctor is using a computer may be longer, and tend to be more doctor focused (Pringle et al., 1986). This latter finding warrants further investigation, given the possible adverse consequence of doctor-focused consultations with patients having a chronic disease requiring active patient management, such as diabetes. In a prospective study of 91 newly diagnosed patients, the majority were distressed about the uncertainties surrounding the nature of the disease at the end of their first year. These uncertainties remained unresolved when a doctor-centred style of communication was used (Mason, 1985). As with patients, it is likely that doctors will vary in their attitudes to the use of information technology in the consultation; this may influence the effect that their use of it has upon their patients.

For both doctors and patients the continuing developments within a field serve to encourage optimism, particularly in the face of a chronic and seemingly intractable problem, such as diabetes. Feeling hopeful may have several benefits, such as encouraging people to continue their efforts with daily management aimed at keeping blood glucose levels close to normal. It may also promote mood states that positively affect physiological functioning

(Totman, 1990).

The other side of this coin is the false raising of hope, the encouragement of certainty when there is none. While uncertainty is inherent in the subject matter of medicine, as well as life, medical education generally does not equip doctors to deal with it and may present a discipline characterised by certainty (Atkinson, 1984). Light (1979) argued that doctors overcome the discomfort of uncertainty by adopting certain strategies, including control over their relationship with the patient, and a tendency to emphasize treatment procedures and techniques, and play down the uncertain nature of the outcome. It is possible that new technology may be used to lessen the uncertainty inherent in many clinical situations.

While new developments may sustain hope and maintain flagging motivation, there is a danger that they may deflect attention from more difficult but ever present issues. In diabetes, these may be the unrelenting daily practical management of the disease. CSII pumps hold the potential for improved flexibility of diabetic regimens without compromising control. At the same time, however, their effective use depends upon assiduous monitoring of blood glucose levels. Bradley and colleagues (1987) in their evaluation of CSII pumps reported that doctors referred to pumps as though they control blood glucose levels, thereby minimising the part that the patient plays. Patients using CSII pumps, who experienced episodes of ketoacidosis, differed from those who did not in feeling less personally in control of their diabetes, perceiving outcomes as less foreseeable, and attributing more responsibility for diabetes management to treatment (Bradley et al., 1986). The authors suggested that over optimistic expectations of this new technology may have encouraged patients to assume that less personal responsibility for their diabetes was required of them than with injection treatment.

The presence of new technology may also distract attention away from the high likelihood that the outcome hoped for will not be achieved. For example, highly technical infertility treatment, such as invitro-fertilisation has a reported success rate of about 10%. This low probability of success and the likelihood that a couple will remain infertile is not highlighted; maybe patients and staff need high hopes to continue with a difficult and stressful procedure against the odds of success (Johnston et al., 1987). In diabetes, the goal of overcoming complications using latest technology may inhibit acknowledgement and discussion of the more pressing reality of the possibility of diabetic complications.

Staff and Patient Training

The introduction of new technology happens in waves. It is introduced by innovators and then taken up by others. While innovators will have high levels of knowledge and expertise in using the technologies, the majority of staff who subsequently use the technologies will not. Unless transfer is planned, staff at the second stage of diffusion may lack the knowledge to implement the new technology effectively. There is a tendency for patients and health professionals to assume uniformly high levels of expertise in health professionals. However, even basic knowledge about diabetes management when assessed has been found lacking (Etzwiler, 1967; Scheiderich *et al.,* 1983; Cumins *et al.,* 1983; Smith & Funnell, 1984). Staff are frequently expected to implement new techniques without adequate knowledge. In one study it was found that 45% of midwives presenting a screening test for a fetal abnormality to pregnant women lacked even basic knowledge about the test (Sanden, 1985). Training of staff will remove one important source of error in patients' use of new techniques (Marteau & Johnston, 1990).

Summary and Conclusions

New advances are rarely uniformly good: they invariably involve costs as well as benefits. All new technologies need to be evaluated fully and evaluation should include psychological as well as physiological predictors and outcomes. In this way it is possible to determine what is effective and for whom (Bradley, 1988). Development of a new technique is just the beginning of the story: its effectiveness depends critically upon consideration of patients' as well as staff's attitudes and behaviour. Awareness of barriers to, and adverse consequences from, use of new technologies for patients, as well as health professionals, can facilitate more effective implementation.

The rapid and increasing development of new technologies in health care presents new challenges for doctors, patients and their relationship. Meeting these challenges is likely to have benefits for both patients and doctors in achieving outcomes from a shared venture.

References

Atkinson, P. (1984). Training for uncertainty. *Social Science and Medicine* 19, 949–956
Bandura, A. (1977. Towards a unifying theory of behaviour change. *Psychological Review* 84, 191–215
Baum, M., Zalkha, K. and Houghton, J. (1989). Ethics of clinical research: lessons for the future. *British Medical Journal* 299, 251–253
Bradley, C., Gamsu, D.S., Knight, G., Boulton, A.J.M. and Ward, J.D. (1986). Predicting risk of diabetic ketoacidosis in patients using continuous subcutaneous insulin infusion. *British Medical Journal* 293, 242–243
Bradley, C., Gamsu, D.S., Moses, J.L., Knight, G., Boulton, A.J.M., Drury, *et al.* (1987). The use of diabetes-specific perceived control and health belief measures to predict treatment choice and efficacy in a feasibility study of continuous subcutaneous insulin infusion pumps. *Psychology and Health* 1, 133–146
Bradley, C. (1988). Clinical trials – Time for a paradigm shift? *Diabetic Medicine* 5, 107–109

Brehm, S.W. (1956). Post-decisional changes in desirability of alternatives. *Journal of Abnormal and Social Psychology* **52**, 384–389

Brownbridge, G., Herzmark, G.A. and Wall, T.D. (1985). Patient reactions to doctors' computer use in general practice consultations. *Social Science and Medical* **20**, 47–52

Council for Science and Society (1982). *Expensive Medical Technology*. London

Cruickshank, P.J. (1982). Patient stress and the computer in the consulting room. *Social Science Medicine* **16**, 1371–1376

Cumins, A.G., Knight, P.V. and Kesson, C.M. (1983). Is ignorance of diabetes mellitus confined to patients alone? Proceedings of the BDA Medical and Scientific Section. Spring Meetings, April, 1983

Davies, A.G., Price, D.A., Houlton, C.A., Burn, J.L., Fielding, B.A., Postlethwaite, R.J. (1984). Continuous subcutaneous insulin infusion in diabetes mellitus. *Archives of Disseases of Childhood* **57**, 1027–33

Deadman-Spall, J.M., Owens, R.G., Leinster, S.J., Slade, P.D. and Dewey, M.J. (1990). Exercising control in treatment choice for breast cancer – does it help? The British Psychological Society Abstracts, p.33

Etzwiler, D.D. (1967). Who's teaching the diabetic? *Diabetes* **16** 111–117

Fallowfield, L. (1988). Controversy over mammographic screening. *British Medical Journal* **297**, 1266–1267

Fallowfield, L.J., Hall, A., Maguire, G.P. and Baum, M. (1990). Psychological outcomes of different treatment policies in women with early breast cancer outside a clinical trial. *British Medical Journal* **301**, 575–80

Festinger, L. and Carlsmith, J.M. (1959). Cognitive consequences of forced compliance. *Journal of Abnormal and Social Psychology*. **58**, 203–210

Fischoff, B. (1982). For those condemned to study the past: Heuristics and biases in hindsight. In: D. Kahneman, P. Slovic and A. Tversky (Eds.). *Judgement under Uncertainty: Heuristics and Biases*. (pp.335–51). New York: Cambridge University Press

Greenfield, S., Kaplan, S.H. and Ware, J.E. (1985). Expanding patient involvement in care. *Annals of Internal Medicine* **102**, 520–528

Greenfield, S., Kaplan, S.H., Ware, J.E. Yano, E.M. and Frank. H.J.L. (1988). Patients' participation on medical care: Effects on blood sugar control and quality of life in diabetes. *Journal of General Internal Medicine* **3**, 448

Johnston, K. (1989). Screening for cervical cancer: A review of the literature. Health Economics Research Unit discussion paper (04/89). Aberdeen: University of Aberdeen

Johnston, M., Shaw, R.W. and Bird, D. (1987). 'Test-tube baby' procedures: Stress and judgements under uncertainty. *Psychology and Health* **1**, 25–38

Light, D. (1979). Uncertainty and control in professional training. *Journal of Health and Social Behaviour* **20**, 310–322

Lowery, B.J. and DuCette, J.P. (1976). Disease related learning and disease control in diabetics as a function of locus of control. *Nursing Research* **25**, 358–362

McNeil, B.J., Pauker, S.G., Sox, H.C. and Tversky, A. (1982). On the elicitation of preferences for alternative therapies. *New England Journal of Medicine* **306**, 1259–1262

Marteau, T.M. (1989). Psychological costs of screening. *British Medical Journal* **299**, 527

Marteau, T.M. (1989a). Framing of information: its influence upon decisions of doctors and patients. *British Journal of Social Psychology* **28**, 89–94

Marteau, T.M. (1989b). Ethics of clinical research. *British Medical Journal* **299**, 513–514

Marteau, T.M. and Johnston, M. (1990). Health professionals: A source of variance in health outcomes. *Psychology and Health* **5**, 47–58

Marteau, T.M., Johnston, M. Baum, J.D. and Bloch, S. (1987). Goals of treatment in diabetes: A comparison of doctors and parents of children with diabetes. *Journal of Behavioural Medicine* **40**, 33–48

Marteau, T.M. Johnston, M. Wynne, G. and Evans, T.R. (1989). Cognitive factors in the explanation of the mismatch between confidence and competence in performing basic life support. *Psychology and Health* **3**, 173–182

Mason, C. (1985). The production and effects of uncertainty with special reference to diabetes mellitus. *Social Science and Medicine* **21**, 1329–1334

Mazze, R.S., Shamoon, H., Pasmantier, R., Lucido, D. and Murphy, J. (1984). Reliability of blood glucose monitoring by patients with diabetes mellitus. *American Journal of Medicine* **77**, 211–217

Mechanic, D. (1979). *Future issues in health care: Social Policy and The Rationing of Medical Services*. New York: The Free Press

Pringle, M., Robins, S. and Brown, G. (1986). Timer: a new objective measure of consultation content and its application to computer assisted consultation. *British Medical Journal* **293**, 20–22

Pueschel, S.M., Monteiro, L.A. and Erickson, M. (1986). Parents' and physicians' perceptions of facial plastic surgery in children with Down's syndrome. *Journal of Mental Deficiency Research* **30**, 71–79

Rethans, J.J., Hoppener, P., Wolfs, G. and Diederiks, J. (1988). Do personal computers make doctors less personal? *British Medical Journal* **296**, 1446–1448

Roter, D. (1977). Patient participation in the patient-provider interaction: The effects of patient question-asking on the quality of interaction, satisfaction, and compliance. *Health Education Monographs* **5**, 281–330

Royal College of General Practitioners (1980). Computers in primary care: the report of the computer working party. Occasional Paper. *Journal of Royal College of General Practitioners* **13**

Sanden, M.L. (1985). Midwives' knowledge of the alphafetoprotein test. *Journal of Psychosomatic Obstetrics and Gynaecology* **4**, 23–30

Scheiderich, S.D., Freibaum, C.N. and Peterson, L.M. (1983). Registered nurses' knowledge about diabetes mellitus. *Diabetes Care* **6**, 57–61

Smith, S.K. and Funnell, M.M. (1984). Diabetes care skills: analysis of perceived importance and competence of health care professionals. *Diabetes* **33**, 77A

Totman, R. (1990). *Mind, stress and health*. London: Souvenir Press Ltd

Tringo, J.L. (1970). The hierarchy of preference towards disability groups. *The Journal of Special Education* **4**, 295–306

Tymstra, T. (1989). The imperative character of medical technology and the meaning of 'anticipated decision regret'. *International Journal of Technology Assessment in Health Care* **5**, 207–213

Wagener, J.J. and Taylor, S.E. (1986). What else could I have done? Patients' responses to failed treatment decisions. *Health Psychology* **5**, 481–496

Weinstein, N.D. (1982). Unrealistic optimism about susceptibility to health problems. *Journal of Behavioural Medicine* **5**, 441–460

Appropriate Technology for Improving Diabetes Care: The Approach and Catalytic Role of WHO

Kirsten Staehr Johansen

Chief, Quality of Care and Technologies, World Health Organization, Regional Office for Europe, Copenhagen, Denmark.

Introduction

The European region, despite its political, social and economic variety, is largely characterized by adequate coverage of the population with respect to health care facilities and staffing. For this reason, the main direction of the work of the World Health Organization, Regional Office for Europe (WHO/EURO) is towards the development of strategies for improvements in existing health services. This will be achieved by raising the standard of work performed by all partners in the health care process.

A number of WHO/EURO programmes with this orientation has been introduced during the last 10–15 years. Results, expressed in terms of quality criteria, outcome indicators, guidelines and other types of recommendations, have aimed at creating awareness in the national health authorities, health care providers and the medical profession, stimulating them to make improvements. Quality criteria for drinking water, air and food safety, as well as criteria for quality of nursing care, child health, and the management of specific diseases such as diabetes mellitus, can provide guidance for managing and improving health care.

Technology Assessment and Quality of Care

One approach for promoting the development of quality in health care is to identify appropriate technologies and interventions, taking into consideration the patient's point of view as well as the use of resources. In order to achieve this, the European Member States of the World Health Organization have formulated a European strategy for *Health for All* (WHO Regional Office for Europe, 1985) which emphasizes the need for, and commitment to, establishing quality assurance in health care and a systematic comprehensive assessment of technology.

Two targets of this strategy are of particular relevance:

> **Target 31** – By 1990, all Member States should have built effective mechanisms for ensuring quality of patient care within their health care systems.

and

> **Target 38** – Before 1990, all Member States should have established a formal mechanism for the systematic assessment of the use of health technologies and of their effectiveness, efficiency, safety and acceptability while reflecting national health policies and economic restraints.

The objectives of targets 31 and 38 are interrelated and activities aimed at achieving these objectives are essential for the development of quality of care. Links were established to other targets such as: Target 1 – reduction of health inequalities; Target 2 – the promotion of health capabilities; Target 13 – health promotion policy; Target 26 – a system based on primary health care; Target 35 – use of health information systems. A structural reorganization of the WHO/EURO programme resulted in the establishment of the programme: *Quality of Care and Technologies* (QCT) which became functional in 1982/1983.

At this point it is important to state the WHO definition of appropriate technology, which is that it should be:

> scientifically valid;
> adaptable to local needs;
> acceptable both to the user and the recipient; and
> able to be maintained and utilized with available resources.

The methods and mechanisms for technology assessment have to take into consideration the differences between European health-care systems and their effect on health and use of resources for both the patient and the population as a whole.

However, during the last decade it has become apparent that progress in conventional technology assessment activities does not necessarily lead to improvement in health care (WHO Regional Office for Europe, 1986); (WHO Regional Office for Europe, 1989). There are many reasons for this failure or ineffectiveness some of which could be that:

> assessments are carried out too late to have much influence on the dissemination of technologies;
>
> assessments rarely fulfill all evaluation criteria, including technical, clinical, economic, psychosocial and quality of life factors, especially the effect on cost and health status, essential to rational decision-making in health planning;
>
> assessments are rarely conducted with access to all the necessary data;

no feedback mechanisms are assured;

compliance and appropriate use of assessment results could be improved if medical professionals and patients participated more in the data collection process;

only new technologies are assessed – not current technologies.

Although it has been constantly stressed that technology assessments should ideally be prospective and comprehensive, the inclusion of all appropriate variables has been the exception rather than the rule.

With this situation in mind, WHO has sponsored several assessments of technology, one of which will be described in this chapter.

Objectives of the QCT Programme Regarding Diabetes Care

To establish mechanisms for the assessment and assurance of quality of health care by promoting studies and projects aimed at the production of guidelines, criteria and standards, to facilitate the elaboration, adjustment or change of health policies.

To ensure the development and appropriate use of information systems to be used in assessment and improvement of health care.

To coordinate national and international studies in the context of health services research.

To collaborate with non-governmental organizations and national institutions in the field of health technology assessment and to use the results for the development of quality of care.

To identify institutions able to collaborate in the promotion, implementation and development of quality assurance in health-care services.

To organize national and international courses and seminars for the promotion and development of quality assurance and technology assessment concepts and methods.

The QCT programme also addresses such issues as quantity, coverage, accessibility, acceptability, efficiency, effectiveness and alternatives of health services as well as patient and staff satisfaction.

A useful practice in the evaluation process is to study the variations in the provision, utilization and outcome of various health-care practices. This method, although less widely accepted, has become the cornerstone of the QCT work. Such non-experimental outcome studies often produce material useful for improving clinical practices and provide valuable information which can help to define those problem areas needing further research which cannot be evaluated other than through randomized control trials.

QCT Study: Management of Diabetes Mellitus

The demands of managing insulin-dependent diabetes in order to avoid meta-bolic fluctuations and reduce the risk of future complications have been described in an earlier chapter in this book.

A central dilemma of diabetes treatment is whether the benefits of strict blood glucose control, with respect to prevention of delayed complications, outweigh the costs, i.e. increased risk of hypoglycaemia, increased monitor-ing, injecting and restriction of diet.

In 1982 the continuous subcutaneous insulin infusion (CSII) pump was considered the most important invention since insulin for the management of diabetes. The initial assessment of the pump was based on consecutive studies on metabolic control by conventional therapy versus the insulin pump. At the request of WHO's European Member States, a multinational study was organized to evaluate the insulin pump and to compare it with conventional therapy (Staehr Johansen, 1989a).

The use of the insulin pump in diabetes care raised questions of general concern. How acceptable was this form of treatment to the patient? What was the effect on the patient's state of mind and social relationships? What were the anticipated economic gains and losses? Did the treatment actually achieve its objective namely, improved control of blood glucose concentrations?

Insulin pumps operate by continuously infusing low volumes of insulin into the subcutaneous site through a fine-bore delivery system. The delivery rate is increased for meal times. Pumps are battery driven and the rate electronically controlled. Care and control of the pump imposed a new and unfamiliar set of demands on the patient. The usefulness of such a therapy, leaving aside its outcome for the moment, must depend to a large extent upon the patient's response and perception of its effect on their lifestyle. Some may welcome it, others may reject it.

The study was designed as a randomized clinical control crossover study. The common protocol was prepared collaboratively. Insulin-dependent diabetic patients were recruited from clinics in Tirana, Albania; Karlsburg, DDR; Helsinki, Finland; Montpellier/Toulouse, France; Paris, France; Budapest, Hungary; Oslo, Norway; Barcelona, Spain; Sheffield, United Kingdom; Zagreb, Yugoslavia.

In the starting phase, optimized injection therapy was ensured by an initial *run-in* period of stabilization and the optimization of home testing and self-monitoring – a requirement for the insulin pump treatment. Indicators were recorded on clinical and technical issues, but – and this is particularly important – also on cost, well-being and patient factors such as personality measures and psychosocial data, these constituting the minimum data set.

The results may be summarized as follows:

At each centre, a number of patients, ranging from 23 (Budapest) to 315 (Paris), were invited to join the study after a full description was given and written consent obtained. Of those who agreed to enter the trial, in the number of patients found suitable for inclusion, a wide variation was found. Sheffield was remarkable in that, although an unusually high proportion of the subjects invited were recruited, only a small number were retained through to study completion. There was also a wide variation in the proportion of patients who "refused" to participate in the study (defined as those persons found suitable for randomization who later declined the offer). The reasons for rejecting pump treatment also differed. Almost all patients who declined in Albania and Hungary did so because they did not want to accept any added responsibility for their own care. Drop-out rates ranged from nil (Yugoslavia), to very low (Albania, DDR, France, Hungary) to high (Spain and Montpellier).

One centre, which had the greatest difficulty in acquiring diabetic equipment, actually demonstrated better results in reducing complication rates than other technologically well-equipped centres, a result which provoked much interest. Upon investigation, it was discovered that, at this particular centre, great emphasis had been placed on improved management of the disease and patient education. This stimulated other centres to follow suit. In Albania for example, this approach led to very clear results: the reduction of the hospitalization rate by 30%, reduction of the amputation rate, reduction of ketoacidosis and the establishment of a national diabetes programme.

Overall, before the pump study, mean HbA_{1c} had varied from 6.2 to 10.9 (although different methods were used and there was no standardization). Furthermore, a tendency towards a greater incidence of retinopathy when baseline levels of HbA_{1c} rose was discernable.

The economic conclusion which can be drawn from the analysis of data from Albania, the German Democratic Republic, United Kingdom and Yugoslavia is that, in the management of pump-wearing or injection-using patients, the administrative differences in the provision of health services create cost differences without necessarily improving health. An increase in the number of hospital appointments seems to lead to an increase in unplanned hospital visits, that is, longer inpatient pump training programmes do not appear to reduce the use of emergency services. Less frequent but longer visits cost less to the patient, in terms of time and transport, than more frequent shorter visits. It therefore became apparent that, on cost evidence alone, the pump does not bring any new benefits.

The insulin pump study was particularly valuable, not only as a technology assessment, but also as the catalyst for improvements in the quality of diabetes management. It has promoted the concept of education of the patient and self-monitoring and has proved that metabolic control can be improved by means of conventional therapy, in many instances as much as the use of the insulin pump itself.

These results led to strengthened collaboration between WHO, the International Diabetes Federation (IDF) and the European Council for Clinical and Laboratory Standardization (ECCLS).

A study of immediate treatment results such as HbA_{1c} level and rates of late complication manifestation such as blindness, nephropathy and gangrene is being established by WHO and the IDF, for the purpose of examining the state-of-the-art of diabetes care in Europe. This will be the first step towards the goal set by WHO and the IDF of reducing complication rates by 30–50% over the next 5 years (Staehr Johansen, 1989b).

Thus, the issue has outgrown the introduction of the insulin pump to encompass improved diabetes management, outcome and cost-effectiveness through multinational, multidisciplinary collaborative efforts.

This theme was later taken up at the recent joint WHO/IDF Meeting on: *Diabetes Mellitus in Europe: A problem at all ages in all countries – A model for prevention and self care*, held in St. Vincent (Aosta), Italy, 10–12 October 1989 (WHO Regional Office for Europe, 1990). A wide range of topics was covered including: the epidemiology of diabetes and its complications, actions needed for better care, European programmes and experiences, economics and the role of social institutions at national and international levels. Approximately 250 participants from all European Member States attended the meeting, representing politics, industry, diabetic patients, insurance, the medical and nursing professions. The following recommendations were made:

Reduce new blindness due to diabetes by one third or more;

Reduce the number of people entering end-stage diabetic renal failure by at least one third;

Reduce by one half the rate of limb amputations for diabetic gangrene;

Cut morbidity and mortality from coronary heart disease in the diabetic by vigorous programmes of risk factor reduction;

Achieve pregnancy outcome in the diabetic woman that approximates that of the non-diabetic woman.

Establish monitoring and control systems using state-of-the-art information technology for quality assurance of diabetes in health care provision and for laboratory and technical procedures in diabetes diagnosis, treatment and self-management.

Promote European and international collaboration in programmes of diabetes research and development through national, regional and WHO agencies and in active partnership with diabetic patients' organizations.

Take urgent action in the spirit of the WHO programme *Health for All* to establish joint machinery between WHO and the IDF, European Region to initiate, accelerate and facilitate the implementation of these recommendations.

Discussion and Future Perspectives

In this age of turbulent technological change, it becomes ever more crucial that systems of evaluation are created which will be of greatest benefit to the patient. The care of the diabetic patient is one excellent example of the need for such a system of evaluation which, once established, could serve as a model for other diseases.

Technology assessment is a complex process. The process begins with initial agreement as to objectives: the framework is discussed at a later stage. The final agreement on the technology under assessment must be based on facts, which must take into consideration its relevance, acceptability to the patient and medical staff, usefulness and effect on both individual health and the health care system as a whole.

Synthesis characterizes the first stage of the assessment process, when the experts must agree to assess a particular technology and its problems comparatively. At this stage, technology assessment bodies should seek the advice and input of the involved parties before deciding where to invest valuable resources and manpower.

The second stage is to raise the level of information, either by exposing the gap between knowledge and practice or, by commissioning further research. Regardless of the specific method of assessment (series, surveillance, case studies, epidemiological, sample surveys or technical trials), valid and reliable information must be the basis for sound analysis. Technology assessment may use routine data collection to determine outcome and cost of the different approaches under assessment, according to the respective study design and protocol. Therefore, information systems, either manual or computerized are essential to the technology assessment process. Initial agreement on the specific assessment methodology, protocol and evaluation mechanisms, is vital, both for ensuring optimal compliance and deciding ultimate action.

The third stage is to reach agreement on interpretation, conclusions, and mode of dissemination of results. It is WHO's experience that agreement can be reached among the panel of experts from different disciplines if the data are valid. However, it is obvious that international multicentre studies face additional challenges. The national political system has a strong influence on any site's compliance with use of assessment protocols, data submission, and data reliability. However, these obstacles are not necessarily insurmountable. It can be both pragmatic and challenging to translate conclusions into actions appropriate to each country. Furthermore, by spreading a technology assessment study over many sites, the risk of it being only of local application can be counteracted. Data collected from multiple sites allows for comparison of variation of outcome and cost as well as identification of the best performing centres. In order to understand differences in practice, liaison between centres and analysis of best demonstrated practice should be established in order to improve the overall quality of care at all sites.

Unfortunately, all too often, this kind of data analysis is reserved for academic workers and certain specific professions which may be one explanation for the negligible impact that technology assessments have generally had on progress in the quality of health care. Therefore, professional organizations should be encouraged to develop and agree on which guiding quality indicators are acceptable and effective for the practical monitoring and assessment of technologies, particularly those currently in use.

The role of the patient as an expert is crucial though it has its limitations. Patients are usually knowledgable about their own particular case, but less so on the disease or disability as a whole or its impact on the health care system. Nevertheless, patients in their role as consumers, agree that better health outcome and improvement in the quality of health care should be goals for all: patients, professionals, management, insurance bodies, the health care industry and politicians.

If the 38 WHO European targets of the *Health for All* strategy are to be achieved, it is essential that appropriate systems for technology assessment be further developed. It may therefore be necessary to test, evaluate and employ various innovative approaches to technology assessment.

The experience of the Quality of Care and Technologies Programme has removed any doubt as to the value of international cooperation in health service research relative to quality of care. In such research, the participation of specialists and institutions from many countries has a number of advantages some of which are:

creation or development of local expertise in a given area;

  raising of the level of awareness of health authorities or health care providers regarding quality of care issues useful for the planning or review of health policies;

  obtaining widely diverse data of greater validity for planning policies of worldwide application;

  reduction of the time it takes to gather statistics and results as a beneficial result of full cooperation.

A number of difficulties are typically encountered in multinational studies. These are usually due to differences in medical practices, differences in definition of a particular disease, differences in interpretation of the protocol and the accuracy with which questions are translated, answered and recorded. With perserverance, these obstacles can be overcome, the study launched and conclusions reached. As an additional bonus, the experience itself may have helped to improve understanding and international cooperation between experts.

Summary

In the World Health Organization's European strategy for *Health for All*, two specific targets (31 and 38) are programmes for quality assurance and technology assessment respectively: considerable importance is given to the development of strategies for improving the quality of health services and the management of specific diseases, with diabetes proving to be a useful model for dealing with other non-communicable diseases. In the management of such diseases, it is of crucial importance to weigh the benefits introduced by certain specific measures against the costs – this is a central issue in the assessment of continuous subcutaneous insulin infusion (CSII) pump therapy in diabetes.

WHO and the International Diabetes Federation have jointly issued a policy statement on the future of diabetes management in Europe ("The St. Vincent Declaration") which includes recommendations for reduction of the complications of diabetes; establishment of monitoring, control and education systems; and the promotion of national and international research. However experience has shown that, if a diabetes care programme is to be truly effective, it is essential that *all* health care partners (patients, professionals, administration, politicians, insurance bodies and the health care industry) participate and collaborate.

References

WHO Regional Office for Europe (1985). *Targets for health for all*, Copenhagen.

WHO Regional Office for Europe (1986). *Evaluation of the Strategy for Health for all by the Year 2000 – Seventh Report on the World Health Situation, volume 5, European Region*, Copenhagen.

WHO Regional Office for Europe (1989). *Monitoring of the strategy for Health for All by the year 2000: Part 1. The situation in the European Region, 1987/88, Copenhagen.*

WHO Regional Office for Europe (1990). *Diabetes Mellitus in Europe: A problem at all ages in all countries – A model for prevention and self care.* Report on a meeting organized jointly by the Regional Office for Europe, World Health Organization and the International Diabetes Federation, European Region, St. Vincent, Italy, 10–12 October 1989, Copenhagen.

Staehr Johansen, K., (1989a). *World Health Organization Multicentre Continuous Subcutaneous Insulin Infusion Pump Feasibility and Acceptability Study Experience.* WHO Regional Office for Europe, Copenhagen.

Staehr Johansen, K., (1989b). Diabetes Management. *International Hospital Federation Yearbook.* Hospital Management International, 96–98.

5

EVALUATION OF NEW TECHNOLOGIES

The World Health Organisation perspective on technology development, described in Kirsten Staehr Johansen's chapter in the previous section, emphasised the importance of measuring psychological and economic outcomes if new technologies are to be evaluated and used appropriately. In this section the focus is directed towards the psychological and economic factors in the evaluation process. The first chapter by Clare Bradley considers the importance of measuring psychological factors when conducting clinical trials of new technologies, not only so that psychological outcomes can be assessed but also to allow consideration of the psychological processes involved in determining effectiveness of treatment and individual differences in treatment outcomes. In particular it is recognised that unless patients' preferences are considered when recruiting patients into a trial and in allocating patients to treatment, the assumptions of the conventional randomised controlled trial design are likely to be undermined and motivational factors will distort the findings. The advantages of alternative designs are discussed. Other chapters, notably the chapters by Marteau and by Gillespie also review research concerned with the study of psychological processes such as health beliefs, perceived control and knowledge of diabetes and their role in determining response to new treatments for diabetes, screening and monitoring procedures. With the increasing interest in psychological outcomes and processes our understanding of the reasons for variation between technologies and between users of the technologies will increase. This will improve the effectiveness and acceptability of new technologies while clinicians can be better advised how they in turn can best advise individual patients.

Recently there have been considerable advances made in the development of scales to measure psychological outcomes and psychological processes. The chapter by Keith Meadows is specifically concerned with the measurement of the psychological outcome of interest to all researchers in the field, quality of life. Following a discussion of the problems of defining and measuring quality of life and assessing the reliability and validity of newly constructed measures, Meadows reviews the instruments that have already been developed to measure certain aspects of the quality of life of people with diabetes. These measures are available to researchers wanting to evaluate the impact of a new technology on the quality of life of the patient users as well as on their metabolic control.

Our final chapter by John Brazier and Richard Jeavons addresses the issue of economic evaluation, an essential aspect of any evaluation of new technologies in diabetes management. The complexity of interrelationships between economic and psychological factors is considered both with respect to doctors' and patients' behaviour concerning diabetes management. The authors point out that despite the methodological and practical problems, economic evaluation...

> "knows its own limitations as a decision aiding technique and makes the necessary value judgements in decision making more explicit. In doing so, it forces us to consider ethical questions about whose values count, the interdependence of individuals' well being and the potential conflict between individual and collective interest."

Similarly one of the spin offs from developing instruments to measure quality of life is that the researchers concerned make explicit their definitions, assumptions and value judgements, in a way that clinicians rarely do. Reliability and validity of newly designed measures are studied and the limitations of the measures are explicitly considered. In choosing between available measures, medical researchers are invited to consider their own assumptions and value judgements. If medical researchers work with psychologists and economists from the design stage of studies for evaluating new technologies in diabetes management, or better still they collaborate from the very first stages of conceptualising the new technology, the perspectives of all are likely to be broadened, and understanding of each others' specialist language, concepts and methods will be likely to increase. This book represents one attempt to facilitate the convergence of the different perspectives and encourage greater efforts at multidisciplinary collaboration in the future.

Evaluating New Technologies: Psychological Issues in Research Design and Measurement

Clare Bradley

Joint appointment between Department of General Practice, UMDS, Guy's Campus, London Bridge, London SE1 9RT and Department of Psychology, Royal Holloway and Bedford New College, Egham Hill, Egham, Surrey TW20 0EX, UK.

New technology needs to be properly evaluated if it is not to be inappropriately advocated or inappropriately discarded. In this chapter it is argued that proper evaluation of new technologies for diabetes care requires that psychological issues be considered. Evaluation studies are rarely designed with a view to measuring or controlling for psychological variables. The physician may focus on the particular needs of the individual patient in the consulting room, when that patient's preferences, motivations, lifestyle and priorities are often considered in deciding treatment regimens and in solving problems with diabetes control but in the context of a study evaluating a new form of technology the focus changes. The study is designed and the data analysed with a view to answering a question which, typically, is something like 'Is this new treatment useful in improving the blood glucose control of Type 1 diabetic patients?'. The individuals disappear. Psychological variables disappear. From such a study the physician aims to determine the effects of a treatment on metabolic control not in individual patients, but in a group of patients.

The fate of new technologies is usually decided on the strength of such studies. For those technologies which survive such evaluation, the physician is then faced with the task of advising an individual patient about the pros and cons for that individual of using the new technological aid to diabetes management, equipped only with information about medical outcomes averaged over groups of selected patients. Such information is not very helpful in predicting whether the new treatment will suit the needs of the particular individual in the consulting room. In this chapter I will consider the origins of the most commonly used form of clinical trial design, the randomised controlled trial, then elaborate further on earlier arguments against the use of standard randomised controlled trial designs and in favour of alternative designs (Bradley, 1988; Brewin and Bradley, 1989). These arguments will be applied in considering the problems of evaluating the use of new technologies for diabetes management.

Early Resistance to Clinical Trials

It is interesting to note that as recently as the late 1940's the great majority of the medical establishment viewed with deep foreboding the idea of applying scientific methods to the evaluation of medical treatments. The randomised controlled trial was regarded with distrust by many who resisted any change from the traditional methods which relied on clinical experience. Indeed, despite the importance and influence of Cochrane's (1972) book on effectiveness and efficiency, which put randomised controlled clinical trials on the map in the early seventies, the influence of the controlled clinical trial was still not universal. Armstrong (1977) provided an anthology of quotes from early opponents to randomised controlled trials to indicate the nature of their worries about scientific methods replacing clinical observation as the main source of data for comparing treatments. The fears expressed in the 1940s may be seen to have some foundation when we consider the way that randomised controlled trials tend to be used today. There were three sets of fears expressed which can be summarised as follows:

1. Scientific trials would be inhumane;
2. Scientific trials would ignore individual differences;
3. Scientific trials would be misleading.

The first fear was essentially that patients would not be considered as people in clinical trials. Grieve (1945) was concerned that,

> 'Medicine ... must have its philosophers if the patients are to be treated as human beings and not as a series of laboratory exercises',

and later wrote,

> 'In our scientific quest let us ever remember that presently much neglected part of man, his soul, has a right to consideration as well as the mechanics of his feet or the biochemistry of his brain' (Grieve, 1946).

We should remember that currently much neglected aspect of humans, their psyche, not least because that psyche will have a powerful influence on the mechanics of the feet and on the biochemisty of the brain. Psychological processes and outcomes are rarely considered in clinical trials and yet can be crucial determinants of medical outcomes.

The fear that scientific trials would ignore individual differences was summed up by Ambrose (1950) in the simple observation, made with reference to the use of antihistamine in the treatment of the common cold and in protest against findings of a Medical Research Council trial, 'Some people do respond and others do not'. Differences which are important and meaningful are frequently relegated to the status of noise in the pursuit of a straightforward answer. Moynihan (1930), in an address published in the Lancet, wrote that the great advances resulting from clinical observation were 'disparaged and in danger of being forgotten. The method of experiment has captured the fancy of many members of our profession, and by reason of the precision of its facile results has created a degree of confidence which has never attached itself to clinical observation alone'.

This very phenomenon which Moynihan described can be seen in studies involving continuous subcutaneous insulin infusion (CSII) pumps (externally worn pumps for the continuous delivery of insulin) where researchers have hoped to answer the question 'Do CSII pumps control blood glucose levels better than injections?' without recognising that neither pumps nor injections can operate independently of the active involvement of the individual using them. Where I depart from Moynihan is with the view he expressed about the problem of individual differences in response to treatments:

'The very complexity of the problem renders it impossible to consider alongside the methods of the laboratory. In hominal research we are able to control only a few specific features; the majority are altogether beyond our control, unapproachable and immutable.'

While it may be difficult to consider the complexities of individual differences between patients, it is not impossible. Psychological differences are perhaps among the most complex of individual differences yet psychological factors can certainly be measured and investigated using scientific methods. Individual differences can be a focus of study but they rarely are.

Towards More Meaningful Clinical Trials

Lack of concern with psychological factors and with individual differences generally can lead to highly misleading conclusions. New treatments may be inappropriately discarded or inappropriately advocated because:

a. metabolic outcomes were the only outcomes considered and/or
b. the treatments were evaluated on groups of patients selected according to inappropriate selection criteria, and benefits or harmful consequences to individuals were ignored.

Consideration of Psychological as well as Metabolic Outcomes

In a randomised controlled trial of a new treatment compared with a conventional treatment, metabolic outcomes may be no better than with conventional treatment although psychological outcomes may well have shown benefits if they had been measured. Conversely metabolic outcomes may indicate significant advantages over conventional treatment while psychological outcomes may have shown unwanted damaging consequences of the new treatment. In clinical trials of CSII, metabolic outcomes typically suggest that

CSII should not be offered because it is not associated with any better blood glucose control than can be achieved using multiple injection therapy and multiple injection therapy is cheaper (eg Marshall *et al.*, 1987). Psychological outcomes, on the other hand, have suggested that CSII should be offered. In a feasibility study in Sheffield where patients with Type 1 diabetes were offered the choice of CSII, intensified conventional treatment, or conventional treatment, it was found that although improvements in glycaemic control were similar for patients using CSII and for those using intensified injection regimens, only the group of patients using CSII reported a significant improvement in their satisfaction with treatment (Lewis *et al.*, 1988).

In the ideal world there is no reason why psychological outcome measures should not always be included in clinical trials evaluating new treatments. In reality, such trials are usually designed by medical personnel who typically do not have the knowledge or experience of dealing with psychological constructs and their measurement. However, in recent years there has been a growing interest in measuring subjective experience of health, psychological well-being and quality of life. The lack of readily available reliable and valid psychological outcome measures has often been given as the reason why such outcomes were not measured and policy decisions were based on clinical judgement supported only by measures of metabolic and clinical outcomes.

Psychologists have until recently found difficulty in persuading funding bodies to give the development of such measures sufficient priority. It is interesting to note that despite the increased availability of measures of psychological outcomes over the past few years there remains a good deal of anxiety and suspicion about the reliability and validity of these measures (often called 'soft'measures) which are unfamiliar to physicians. Meanwhile biochemical measures with which clinicians are only too familiar (often called 'hard' measures) are accepted without a second thought, glycosylated haemoglobin being a common example (Home, 1990). Concern is expressed that, for example, psychological outcomes may be influenced by such factors as the weather, with warm summer days being associated with more positive affect than cold winter days. How can we use an outcome measure that is so susceptible to external influence? The knowledge that weight and blood glucose control also vary with the seasons is curiously often ignored, such measures commonly being used without thought for their reliability and validity. Koran (1975a and b) reviewed what little evidence was available on the reliablity of clinical methods and data and showed that there were no grounds for complacency. It may be hoped that one of the spin offs of medical researchers learning to assess the reliability, validity and suitability of psychological outcome measures for clinical trials may be that they come to reassess other more familiar and taken-for-granted measures. They may come to recognise that these so-called 'hard' measures often have soft centres.

A variety of psychological outcome measures is now available and more are being developed. Papers describing the development of such measures now appear in clinical medical journals (eg Bradley and Lewis, 1990;

Nicassio *et al.*, 1985) and are thus being brought to the attention of physicians directly rather than via their social science colleagues. McDowell and Newell (1987) have compiled a useful guide to scales and questionnaires for measuring health. This guide is a valuable tool for researchers trying to find a suitable off-the-peg measure though it should be borne in mind that scales developed on non-diabetic populations may not be appropriate for people with diabetes. The chapter by Meadows in the present volume considers how psychological outcomes can be measured. Here I simply illustrate the need to measure such outcomes if a realistic evaluation of a treatment is to be made.

Consideration of Individual as well as Group Differences

When focusing on groups of patients the researcher attempts to answer the question 'Which treatment is best for this population as a whole?' It could be that in a randomised controlled trial comparing two treatments, half the patients allocated to the new treatment do exceptionally well and half allocated to the conventional treatment do exceptionally well, so that the researcher concludes there is no difference between the treatments. The group focus suggests that there is no advantage in offering the new treatment although for individual patients this may be quite untrue. It may make a great deal of difference to their psychological and metabolic well-being if they can have the choice of treatment. Randomised controlled trials are not incompatible with an individual focus though in practice most randomised controlled trials have an exclusively group focus. Individual differences are not usually considered or analysed and where they are, only metabolic/ clinical variables are usually considered.

Choice of Appropriate Selection Criteria and Recruitment Procedures

If we investigate demographic and psychological variables to see which kind of patients benefit from a treatment and which do not benefit then we can gather systematic data about the appropriateness of the selection criteria in that particular trial. At present, however, while scientific principles may guide the design of a clinical trial, the selection criteria are determined by such factors as clinical judgement and unsubstantiated beliefs about what kind of people will be suitable, or, by criteria used in an earlier study and unthinkingly applied again.

Selection criteria which superficially appear to be simple and straightforward may sometimes mask a multitude of complex psychological factors that may influence supposedly clinical variables in ways that go unrecognised. An example is provided in a review of implantable insulin pumps (Selam, 1988) where two studies were described as 'very comparable in terms of ...patient selection' yet the selection criteria were simply 'CSII treated Type 1 diabetes of long duration'. The comparability of the two studies of implantable pumps will therefore depend on the selection criteria used in allocating CSII which may or may not be very comparable. We need to know what the patients were told about CSII, what they expected from CSII and why they thought that the treatment might suit them. Sometimes the patient may simply have followed the advice of their doctor that CSII was the best treatment even though remaining sceptical about the suitability of the treatment for themselves.

In the Sheffield feasibility study of CSII versus conventional treatments, patients were recruited into the study with a talk on the three treatment options. They were told among other things that 'the evidence suggests that CSII pumps will control your blood sugar better than injections'. Before any changes were made to the treatment regimen patients in this study completed a series of psychological measures including a scale to measure Perceived Control over diabetes. It was found that the patients who chose the pumps were more likely to be those with a stronger sense of Medical Control over their diabetes (ie those attributing diabetes-related outcomes to the medical staff and the treatment prescribed). Those with a stronger sense of Personal Control over their diabetes (believing in their personal responsibility and control over outcomes) were not more likely to choose to use CSII (Bradley et al., 1987). The patients most likely to opt for CSII were those who were looking for a medical solution to their diabetes but they had been misled. The CSII pump is only as good at controlling blood glucose levels as its owner enables it to be. The patients with the highest sense of Medical Control among the CSII users turned out to benefit the least from the pump. They had higher HbA_1 levels after 12 months of treatment indicating worse blood glucose control (Bradley et al., 1987) and they were more likely to experience diabetic ketoacidosis while using CSII (Bradley et al., 1986).

The Sheffield study was described as a feasibility study. Patients chose their treatment group. They were not allocated at random. The interaction between the recruitment procedures chosen by the doctors and the beliefs and preferences of the patients became clear in this study where the factors influencing patients' choices were a focus of the investigation. Randomised controlled trials cannot offer immunity from the effects of patients' preferences and beliefs. It is usually assumed that random allocation is the best way of arriving at two similar groups of patients but when patients' reasons for participating in the trial and their preferences for treatments are considered, the justification for this assumption is called into question.When patients agree to participate in a clinical trial a problem arises if that is the only chance that they have of using a new form of treatment (Bradley, 1988). If patients recruited into the study all believe they will prefer the new treatment under evaluation to the conventional comparison treatment (patients preferring the other treatment having chosen it outside of the clinical trial), random allocation of patients to treatment is likely to lead to one group being disappointed with the treatment allocated and another group that is not. The problem is illustrated in Figure 1 where patients in the two treatment groups develop differences following randomisation. These may include differences in their expectations of treatment outcome, enthusiasm for participating in the study, tolerance of inconvenience or discomfort, all of which are likely to have more to do with whether or not the treatment allocated was the preferred form of treatment than with any pharmacological or physiological effects of the treatments. Similar problems are just as likely to arise in randomised controlled trials where patients are crossed over to two or more treatments as in trials with separate parallel treatment groups. Patients may have greater expectations of one treatment than another, may be more enthusiastic about one leg of the trial than the other and so on. The likelihood of such problems arising depends on the context of the study, including the way in which the treatments were presented, and the patients' reasons for agreeing to participate.

In randomised controlled trials, all patients recruited have to be prepared to use any of the treatments being studied. In such trials of CSII versus intensified conventional treatments which were carried out before CSII became more routinely available, it is likely that many if not all patients agreed to

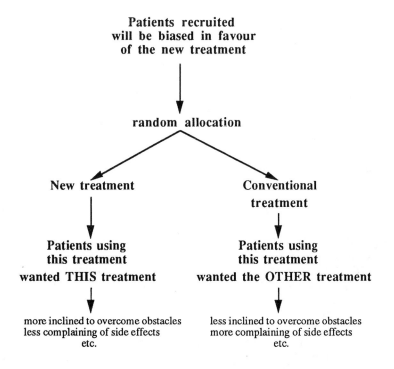

Figure 1. The problem of random allocation creating differences between groups, in trials involving a new treatment which is only available within the trial.

participate in the study because they thought that they would prefer to use CSII. Because CSII was not routinely available, the only opportunity they had to try CSII was by agreeing to the randomization. Those patients who were not prepared to have their treatment allocated at random were not studied. Typically, patients declining to take part in such studies have been the far greater proportion of those invited to participate (Grimm *et al.*, 1987). Unless baseline data are collected on the subjects who decline to take part in the randomised controlled trial, the researchers and everyone else will remain ignorant of the non-representativeness of the sample being randomised.

In summary, there are two problems which usually go unnoticed but may have profound implications for the results of a study and the conclusions about the value of a new treatment. First, randomisation is intended to ensure that differences between the groups not due to intervention are equalised but in this context may actually cause differences in the groups being compared. Secondly, those patients who agree to participate in the study may not be representative of the population as a whole. The conclusions may then be misleading and cannot be generalised. One possible approach to dealing with these problems is matching patients on motivational criteria.

Matching Patients on Motivational Criteria

In theory we could match patients randomised to each treatment group on motivational criteria if we recruited into the trial only those patients who were equally prepared to use any of the treatments involved. In practice this would be likely to be difficult, especially if the treatments were very different. For example, it is hard to imagine that any patient would be equally prepared to use any of the three treatments in the Sheffield CSII feasibility study (CSII, intensified conventional treatment, or conventional treatment). Furthermore, if there were any such willing patients they would be unlikely to be representative of potential users of any one of the treatments alone. We might allocate patients to the treatment of choice rather than on a random basis as was done in the Sheffield feasibility study and explore the factors determining preferences, though the patients in each treatment group will differ on numerous other criteria and differences between groups must be interpreted with great care. Brewin and Bradley (1989) suggested an alternative design which may offer the best of both randomised controlled trial and non-randomised feasibility study designs.

A part-randomised, part-patient-preference-determined design

Brewin and Bradley's (1989) suggested alternative to randomised control trial and non-randomised feasibility study designs will here be applied to a hypothetical study to evaluate glucose sensors; the development of which is described by Pickup in this book. Pickup points out that glucose sensors will not benefit all patients, and cautions that they should not be used indiscriminately. Glucose sensor technology, especially if it were linked to an alarm to signal hypoglycaemia, would be particularly useful for those patients who have lost the warning symptoms of hypoglycaemia (see chapter by Hepburn and Frier). For such individuals, the advantages of a device that allows them to avoid the dangers and embarrassments of unpredictable episodes of unconsciousness might be expected to outweigh the disadvantages of wearing the device. However, for people who have adequate warning symptoms of hypoglycaemia, a glucose sensor would offer less obvious advantage, and the disadvantages would be likely to be more annoying in the absence of any clear benefits. It would be possible to describe a subsample of the diabetic population for whom glucose sensors are anticipated to be useful from which individuals would be recruited into studies evaluating the new technology. Certain objective criteria for recruitment could be set out, such as evidence of hypoglycaemic unawareness, or a history of night time hypoglycaemic reactions. However, not all patients with hypoglycaemic unawareness or recurrent hypoglycaemia will be prepared to use glucose sensors and some may prefer to continue to use intensive blood glucose monitoring even if this means tolerating more hypoglycaemic episodes rather than wear a glucose sensor device. Other patients may be prepared to try glucose sensors but have not tolerated intensive blood glucose monitoring.

Figure 2 illustrates Brewin and Bradley's design which would accommodate patients with a preference for one of the two treatments to be compared, as well as patients with no particular preference. Those patients with a preference for one or other form of treatment would be allocated their preferred treatment. Those patients with no preference would be allocated a treatment at random. Thus there would be a maximum of four treatment groups for study. Groups 3 and 4 would be the nearest equivalent to groups formed in randomised controlled trials with two advantages over those of a standard randomised controlled trial. First, patients in the two groups could be expected to be equivalent in terms of their motivation to use the treatments to which they were allocated at random. The second advantage is that the study would not exclude patients who did have a preference for one of the treatments, but instead would study those patients in one of two separate groups, groups 1 and 2. Comparison of outcomes of group 3 vs group 4 will give us an estimate of the relative value of glucose sensors and blood glucose monitoring for this group of patients where there were no strong preferences to influence the results. Comparison of groups 1 and 3 will give us an estimate of the role of motivational factors in determining the value of glucose sensors. If outcomes in group 1 are significantly better than outcomes in group 3 then motivational factors can be seen to be important. Similarly, comparison of groups 2 and 4 gives us an estimate of the role of motivational factors in blood glucose monitoring. Comparing all four groups provides yet more useful information. If, for example, groups 1 and 3 who both used glucose sensors had significantly better outcomes than group 4 (who had no initial preference and were randomly allocated blood glucose monitoring) but no better than group 2 who were allocated blood glucose monitoring because of an initial preference, then it might be recommended that in future, those patients who strongly prefer blood glucose monitoring to glucose sensors be provided with blood glucose monitoring but all other patients meeting the selection criteria used in this study should be recommended to use glucose sensors.

It may be that there are no patients who prefer one of the treatments over the other in which case the classic randomised controlled trial will result because there will be no groups 1 and 2. However, the preferences of the patients will have been investigated and the possibilities of such preferences biasing the outcomes will have been excluded. More likely, there will be some patients preferring one treatment but none preferring the other and a three group study would result with only a subset of comparisons possible. More likely still, there would be patients with preferences for each of the treatments and patients without preferences but the numbers of patients in each group would vary considerably. In the event that there were too few patients who had no preference to allow randomisation, the study would be limited to groups 1 and 2 in the manner of a feasibility study and the

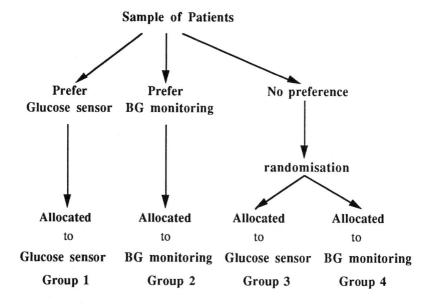

Figure 2. An alternative design to randomised controlled trials for comparing the effects of two treatments, glucose sensors and blood glucose monitoring, while controlling for motivational factors.

conclusions that could be drawn would be limited accordingly. Under this last circumstance of few patients having no preference a variant of this design might be considered whereby half the patients preferring glucose sensors be allocated blood glucose monitoring and half the patients preferring blood glucose monitoring be allocated glucose sensors. Such a design would serve the purpose of controlling for motivational factors though the number of patients willing to be recruited into such a study would be likely to be reduced with a consequent reduction in the representativeness of the sample and would not offer the same advantages as the design portrayed in figure 2.

Since writing the 1989 paper one study has been identified which used such a design to study opiate withdrawal. Gossop *et al.* (1986) assigned patients to inpatient versus outpatient treatment on the basis of strong preference, or randomisation where preference was not strong. Twenty of the sixty subjects studied were willing to accept either in- or out-patient treatment and treatments were allocated to these subjects at random. The forty subjects who expressed a strong preference appeared to be approximately equally divided as to preference for in-patient or out-patient treatment. Thus the study had four groups of adequate size to allow analysis of the data in the manner outlined above. Unfortunately the researchers lost the advantage of the design by combining the groups into in-patient and out-patient samples and testing the significance of differences between these two groups without regard for initial patient preferences and the method of allocation to groups. Thus the design appeared to be employed simply as a device for encouraging subject recruitment into the study rather than as a means of investigating the role of motivational factors in determining treatment efficacy. Fortunately the numbers expressing a preference for each of the treatment options appeared to be evenly distributed (actual numbers were not given and can only be derived approximately). Had the numbers differed substantially, the procedure of combining for analysis randomised and preferred groups would have hopelessly confounded the two variables of preference versus no preference and in- versus out-patient treatment. Whether or not the preferences are evenly distributed the analysis of four separate groups would provide considerably more useful information and is the method of analysis recommended for future studies.

Another researcher who has considered patient preferences is Marteau (1989) who, in the course of pilot work for an evaluation study involving random allocation, investigated patients' preferences for different approaches to preparing them for routine prenatal screening tests (Marteau, 1989). She asked pregnant women if they had a preference for one of the four interventions which were: information to be given

1. in a booklet,
2. during routine antenatal care,
3. at an extra antenatal class or
4. both in a booklet and in an extra class.

Approximately 50% of the women preferred one of the four interventions while 50% had no preference. Preferences were not evenly distributed across the four options. The recruitment procedure was then reconsidered to try and understand why patients were avoiding two of the options (options 1 and 2). The description of the treatment options was modified slightly and the pilot repeated. Preferences were found to be equalised across the four options. These pilot studies suggested that a) we can discover preferences that we did not anticipate if we make a point of investigating preferences, and b) we can sometimes influence patients' preferences very easily with minor changes of wording or emphasis. Several studies are now being planned to use the design suggested by Brewin and Bradley (1989). One study, recently funded by the Scottish Home and Health Department, will evaluate a new method of termination of pregnancy in the first trimester, comparing the new treatment with standard surgical treatment and assigning patients to treatment group according to patient preference, allocating at random only those women who have no preference (Naji, 1990).

In figure 2, the focus was on the issue of patients' preferences and the possibilities of building this variable into the study design. Other ways in which psychological variables might be incorporated into this study have already been addressed earlier in this chapter in other contexts and include

1. the measurement of psychological as well as metabolic outcomes,
2. the investigation of individual differences,
3. determination of selection criteria and recruitment procedures.

If selection criteria are limited to metabolic outcomes it may well be that patients who could benefit from the new technology are not even considered for inclusion in the study. It may be that some patients who have not experienced hypoglycaemic attacks and who have maintained excellent blood glucose control have achieved this only at the expense of considerable personal effort with frequent blood testing, painful fingers and heightened levels of anxiety about the possibility of blood glucose fluctuations which may go unnoticed. Such patients may be motivated to try glucose sensors but the success of the new technology would for them be measured not in terms of improved control and reduced hypoglycaemic episodes, but in terms of improved psychological well-being and satisfaction with the treatment regimen required to attain near-normoglycaemia. If evaluations of new technology exclude such patients, an excellent opportunity to demonstrate the advantages of the technology will be lost. A variety of selection criteria may of course be included, as they often are in clinical practice, and the outcomes associated with the different selection criteria may be investigated in within-group analyses of subgroups of patients.

A range of analyses investigating individual differences would include analyses of the within-group variability in outcomes. Some patients may demonstrate considerable benefits while others in the same treatment group demonstrate no such benefits or even experience unwanted effects from the treatments. Investigation of such differences to try and predict outcomes on the basis of psychological, clinical, metabolic, demographic and other variables measured at the start of the study will be likely to improve our understanding of the processes involved and increase the chances of using the technology appropriately in future. Recruitment procedures are rarely determined, adhered to and described with the same attention to the importance of scientific rigour as are other aspects of clinical trials although recruitment procedures may themselves be regarded as worthy cases for study. In clinical trials which have to settle upon one method of recruitment, pilot work, such as that carried out by Marteau and described above, may be required to determine appropriate procedures for the purposes of that study. Written information for patients being recruited into the study will serve two important purposes; first it will increase the chances of recruiting patients in a uniform fashion and, secondly, the information can be reported verbatim in publications of the study and may be taken into account by readers trying to make sense of differences between the findings of two otherwise apparently similar studies.

Measurement of Psychological Processes

Measures of psychological outcomes are only one subset of psychological measures that should take their place in clinical trials of new technologies in diabetes care. Measures of psychological processes are also important. Without measures of the psychological processes involved all we can do is establish the nature of the outcomes in any particular study. If we are to be able to understand the reasons for the outcomes and increase the chances of improving the outcomes in future studies then we need to include measures of psychological processes. Such measures might include measures of health beliefs and perceptions of control over diabetes which were useful in understanding reasons for different levels of glycaemic control in the patients choosing to use the different treatment options in the Sheffield feasibility study (Bradley *et al.*, 1987), and the reasons for a high incidence of diabetic ketoacidosis among CSII users in that study (Bradley *et al.*, 1986). Other measures that may help to account for individual differences in treatment efficacy, or between-group and between-study differences in outcomes might be measures of patients' knowledge about their diabetes and its treatment, their expectations of the treatments to be evaluated, and measures of the extent to which individuals adhered to the study protocol. With measures such as these and intelligent data analysis we can determine, for example, why glucose sensors are associated with better or worse outcomes than self monitoring of blood glucose. We could better establish the characteristics of the glucose sensor technology, and its use in any particular study, which are responsible for the outcomes obtained. Equipped with such information we would be better able both to improve on glucose sensor technology and to design more appropriate user-friendly technologies in the future.

Summary and Conclusions

Psychological variables need to be considered in

1. measuring outcomes such as patient satisfaction with a new treatment and their psychological well-being for consideration alongside metabolic outcomes in evaluating new technologies in diabetes management,
2. investigating individual differences in expectations of, responses to and outcomes associated with new treatments,
3. determining selection and recruitment criteria,
4. measuring processes such as adherence, knowledge and beliefs with a view to understanding individual and group differences in treatment outcomes.

The psychological variables considered here can indeed be studied with the benefit of scientific methods. Clinical trials which consider and investigate psychological variables may overcome the fears of the early resistance movement against "scientific" clinical trials by becoming more humane, less misleading and more scientific.

References

Ambrose, A.J. (1950). Clinical impression versus cold science. *British Medical Journal* **2**, 631

Armstrong, D. (1977). Clinical sense and clinical science. *Social Science and Medicine* **11**, 599–601

Bradley, C. (1988). Clinical trials – Time for a paradigm shift? *Diabetic Medicine* **5**, 107–109

Bradley, C., Gamsu, D.S., Moses, J.L., Knight, G., Boulton, A.J.M., Drury, J. *et al.* (1987). The use of diabetes-specific perceived control and health belief measures to predict treatment choice and efficacy in a feasibility study of continuous subcutaneous insulin infusion pumps. *Psychol Health* **1**, 133–146

Bradley, C., Gamsu, D.S., Knight, G., Boulton, A.J.M., Ward, J.D. (1986). Predicting risk of diabetic ketoacidosis in patients using continuous subcutaneous insulin infusion. *British Medical Journal* **293**, 242–3

Bradley, C. and Lewis, K.S. (1990). Measures of psychological well-being and treatment satisfaction developed from the responses of people with tablet-treated diabetes. *Diabetic Medicine* **7**, 445–451

Brewin, C.R. and Bradley, C. (1989). Patient preferences and randomised clinical trials. *British Medical Journal* **299**, 313–5

Cochrane, A.L. (1972). *Effectiveness and Efficiency: Random Reflections of Health Services.* The Nuffield Provincial Hospitals Trust

Gossop, M., Johns, A. and Green, L. (1986). Opiate withdrawal: inpatient versus outpatient programmes and preferred versus random assignment to treatment. *British Medical Journal* **293**, 103–104

Grieve, J. (1945). Whither Medicine? *Lancet* **2**, 830–831

Grieve, J. (1946). Whither medicine? *Lancet* **1**, 520

Grimm, J.J., Haardt, M.-J., Thibult, N., Goicolea, I., Tchobroutsky, G., Slama, G. (1987). Lifestyle, metabolic control and social implications of pump therapy in 54 routine Type 1 diabetic patients. *Diabete et Metabolisme* **13**, 3–11

Home, P.D. (1990). Glycosylated haemoglobin revisited. *Diabetic Medicine* **7**, 385–386

Koran, L.M. (1975a). The reliability of clinical methods, data and judgements (first of two parts). *The New England Journal of Medicine* **29**, 642–646

Koran, L.M. (1975b). The reliability of clinical methods, data and judgements (second of two parts). *The New England Journal of Medicine* **29**, 695–701

Lewis, K.S., Bradley, C., Knight, G., Boulton, A.J.M. and Ward, J.D. (1988). A measure of treatment satisfaction designed specifically for people with insulin-dependent diabetes. *Diabetic Medicine* **5**, 235–242

Marshall, S.M., Home, P.D., Taylor, R. and Alberti, K.G.M.M. (1987). Continuous subcutaneous insulin infusion vs injection therapy: a randomised cross-over trial under usual diabetic clinic conditions. *Diabetic Medicine* **4**, 521–525

McDowell, I. and Newell, C. (1987). *Measuring Health: A Guide to Rating Scales and Questionnaires*. New York: Oxford University Press

Marteau, T.M. (1989) Personal communication.

Moynihan, B. (1930). The Science of Medicine. *Lancet* **2**, 779–785

Naji, S. (1990) Personal Communication

Nicassio, P.M., Wallston, K.A., Callahan, L.F., Herbert, M. and Pincus, T. (1985). The measurement of helplessness in rheumatoid arthritis. The development of the Arthritis Helplessness Index. *Journal of Rheumatology* **12**, 462–467

Selam, J.L. (1988). Development of implantable insulin pumps: long is the road. *Diabetic Medicine* **5**, 724–733.

Assessing Quality of Life

Keith A. Meadows

Department of Endocrinology, Charing Cross Hospital, Fulham Palace Road, London W6 8RF and Department of Psychology, Royal Holloway and Bedford New College, Egham Hill, Egham, Surrey TW20 0EX, UK.

Introduction

With the ever growing importance of technology in the management of people with Type 1 (insulin-dependent) diabetes, there is increasing awareness that measurement of physiological outcome is insufficient in the evaluation of benefit to the patient. As a result the measurement of such outcomes as subjective well-being, general health perceptions, functional status and health related quality of life are increasingly recognised as important areas of outcome assessment. The potential of the pen-injector in enabling more freedom in timing of meals and injections, is an example where improvement in the quality of life is paramount.

Recently a plethora of instruments have been used or designed to evaluate the emotional, social, and behavioural aspects of diabetes, many of which can be seen as broadly relating to the concept of quality of life. Regrettably, much of this work lacks a clear theoretical and conceptual framework in its development. Furthermore the instruments have often been developed for use with psychiatric or other illness groups. With attention now increasingly focused on quality assurance, assessment of the patient's quality of life is an intuitively plausable and attractive idea for both groups and individuals.

What is 'quality of life' and how can it be measured? This chapter attempts to discuss some of the main concepts of quality of life in the context of patients with insulin dependent diabetes mellitus.

What do we Mean by Quality of Life?

Quality of life has to do with the individual's experience of living a 'good' or 'bad' life. In discussing the assessment of the goodness or quality of life of an individual, objections will inevitably be raised that such an undertaking is either too philosophically based or unscientific, and therefore not in the realms of scientific research. The information gathered might be subjective and introspective, and therefore unmeasurable.

There is no authoritative statement on what quality of life is, different researchers employing differing terminology. It is often assumed that everyone has an intuitive understanding of the nature of quality of life and that its definition is no more than common sense. However, similar terms including 'well being' and 'satisfaction', also tend to convey to the researcher conceptually similar connotations to 'quality of life' as they are clearly tied to the experiences of the individual. Do they however have the richness and broadness often associated with the meaning of quality of life?

Satisfaction is a precursor to quality of life and much of the research on it has been associated with level of satisfaction in work, occupation and life in general (Neugarten *et al.*, 1961; Liang, 1984; Diener *et al.*, 1985). In diabetes the concept of satisfaction has been tied to patients' perceived satisfaction with medical treatment (Lewis *et al.*, 1988; Bradley and Lewis, 1990). However quality of life must be seen as having a wider frame of reference to include the individual's psychological state as well as social and vocational functioning.

In an attempt to delimitate the concept 'quality of life' Naess (1987) pointed out that some would define the concept narrowly as the predominance of pleasure over pain, whilst others would define it as a basic mood of well-being and contentment. A more extended concept, however, should encompass both the cognitive and affective aspects of the individual's life. The cognitive component should be represented by the assessment of the patient's satisfaction and dissatisfaction with their life situation with respect to the disorder, with expectations and aspirations being major elements. On the other hand the affective aspects should encompass both the positive and negative reactions of the patient, concurrent with the disorder but not necessarily attributable to it. Naess (1987) considers that a person enjoys a high quality of life (or well-being) to the degree that the person

1. is active
2. is able to relate to others
3. has self esteem
4. experiences a basic mood of happiness

Implicit in Naess's definition of quality of life is that the individual's realm of activity would encompass both personal and role functioning and that the level of functioning would be closely related to the physical aspects of the disease, symptoms, pain and emotional responses. Personal functioning could be defined as stated by Ware (1984) as:

> the performance or capacity to perform the kinds of tasks that most people do every day including self-care, mobility and physical activities.

Ware (1984) views role functioning as the performance or capacity of the individual to perform activities associated with employment, school-work, or homemaking.

Naess (1987) considers that these four areas can encompass the most significant aspect of an individual's quality of life with all four areas being afforded equal importance. Similarly, Schipper (1983) considers that in the assessment of the patient's quality of life one needs to focus on day to day aspects of functional living including the psychological, somatic, social and vocational. Wenger (1986) defines quality of life in terms of three main components:

(i)   functional capacity
(ii)   perception of health status
(iii) disease symptoms. The importance of health perceptions or health status as a component in the evaluation of the individual's quality of life was stressed by Ware (1984), in suggesting that its usefulness may lie in the explanation of individual differences in health and illness behaviour.

Operationalizing the Concept of Quality of Life

If the concept of quality of life is to be of any practical value in collecting information on the individuals quality of life it must be translated into operational terms.

A number of studies have considered the impact of illness including cancer and heart disease on the quality of life of patients (Spitzer *et al.*, 1981; Ferrell *et al.*, 1989). However, different illnesses affect different bodily functions leading to different physical and emotional problems. Thus changes in mobility and confinement or leisure and recreational pastimes may be highly salient in patients with rheumatoid arthritis, or changes in body image in patients with breast cancer. How relevant are these issues to the patient with diabetes? Both Schipper (1983) and Guyatt *et al.* (1986) stress that the content of quality of life measures must reflect what is important to the patient. In the operationalization of the concept for diabetes we need to be sensitive to the complexities of the management regimen and the demands it places on the individual patient. To what extent does living with diabetes encroach on the day to day life including work, school, recreational, social, personal and sexual relationships, as well as any impact on the individual's aspirations? We need also to be aware of the patient's own emotional responses and attitudes to diabetes as well as the behaviour and attitudes of others including family, friends and employers. In other words the content needs to reflect 'normal' pursuits and activities. The content however must also take account of whether we are assessing the quality of life of adults, children or adolescents. Recreational pursuits, work activities, career aspirations, peer group pressures etc are all likely to have differing levels of relevance dependent on the stage of life of the patient. It is also advocated in the light of the preceeding discussion that the definition of quality of life should be represented as a multi-dimensional concept covering at least the following four domains of human life.

(i) Psychological State

The assessment of the patient's psychological state is of primary importance because of its effect on the patient's overall well-being and consequently quality of life.

The assessment of psychological state should include both cognitive and affective aspects, through assessments of satisfaction or dissatisfaction with either life in general or specific life situations as a result of diabetes, as well as emotional, positive and negative reactions including depressed mood, feelings of anxiety, hostility and hopelessness. Such reactions should not be seen as representing clinically defined levels of affective disorder, but rather as changes in levels of mood as a possible consequence of living with the disease. Content reflecting somatic symptoms should be selected which is as unconfounded as possible with diabetic symptomatology (such as fatigue). It is important to remember that the emotional state of the patient can be altered by the disease and its treatment. However assessment of psychological state in its own right is necessary, because it will not always correspond to changes in the social or vocational functioning of the patient or physical well-being brought about by treatment intervention.

(ii) Role Functioning

Role functioning should include a number of components which focus on the performance or capacity of the individual in performing 'normal' activities including employment, school work and homemaking. Ware (1984) considers the patient's level of role functioning as a reflection of the patient's health status and the demands of the various role activities of that individual. However the health status of the individual including the physical limitations resulting from the disease will not always affect the role functioning of the individual, but instances of role dysfunction in the absence of physical limitations can often be observed. Thus role dysfunctioning may be brought about by the patient's own perceptions of the illness such as the requirements of the management regimen, anxieties associated with hyper-hypo-glycaemia or simply insufficient diabetes- related knowledge. Therefore the content of this domain should be based on restrictions in life style, and satisfaction in meeting vocational aspirations, but should not be directly related to the physical limitations brought about by the disease.

(iii) Social Support

Social support may modify the impact of illness on the patient (Cohen and Wills, 1985; Schafer et al., 1986; Ganster and Victor, 1988). Therefore it is

H

useful to assess the interpersonal relations of the patient including the presence or absence as well as the quality of a reciprocal relationship with at least one other person, in respect of the management of the disease.

(iv) Physical Well-being

It is also useful to assess the impact of the patient's physical well-being on quality of life due either to acute or chronic limitations in role functioning. This should focus on pertinent physical aspects of the disease including fatigue, symptoms of unstable blood glucose control, impaired vision, and painful peripheral neuropathy. Both the demographic characteristics and disease state of the patients studied should be considered when assessing physical well-being as it can be confounded by medical factors associated with age for example, and the impact of complications at early and later stages of the disease.

Methodological Issues in the Assessment of Quality of Life

In addition to the major issues of defining and operationalizing the concept, there are a number of methodological issues to be considered in the development of a measure of quality of life. Some of these have been discussed briefly by Schipper (1983). These include the need for measures not only to be comprehensive in adequately evaluating the relevant components of quality of life, but also to be sufficiently compact to enable repeated use if necessary. It is important however that both reliability and validity of the measure should not be sacrificed at the expense of producing an instrument appealingly short in completion time and scoring due to restricted content. Furthermore each of the individual components of the measure must be meaningful to all patients. To achieve this the content of the individual components need to be general rather than specific. Quality of life for one patient may be impaired because diabetes restricts visits to friends or relatives and another because dietry restrictions limit eating out. Thirdly the measure must be sensitive enough to detect changes in the quality of life to allow initiation of new interventions when appropriate, and to assess the effects of previous interventions. A further issue is the difficulty in comparing the quality of life between patients. Does the baseline quality of life between a housewife differ from that of a working mother with a similar illness? The problem here is the individual's frame of reference and life experiences. The individual's frame of reference may be a certain group of other people such as workmates, family members, and acquaintances. What the individual is probably expressing is the belief that quality of life is high or low in respect to this frame of reference. Also the individual may also make comparisons with themselves at other times. Perception that circumstances are better now than a year ago will cause a report that quality of life is higher, even if one is less happy than another person who believes and reports a rather low quality of life. Schipper's (1983) approach to this problem of baseline measurement is that measures of quality of life be designed in which the individual patients serve as their own internal controls. This approach places less emphasis on baseline scores and more on the trend in scores over time. As a consequence questions should be designed to elicit answers which are relative in nature ('very much more', 'less satisfactory'). This approach concurs with the notion that the measurement of quality of life is considered as an outcome of the disease and its treatment and that only those aspects of quality of life subject to change over time should be considered relevant.

Finally, we must establish the reliability and validity of the measure of quality of life. As already pointed out the design or selection of an appropriate measure is often lacking in methodological rigour, a prerequisite if quality of life and its measurement are to be credible. As Schipper (1983) rightly points out...

> To rush a half baked index into unfettered clinical use risks discrediting the entire effort.

The measure must possess both reliability and validity. Reliability is evidence that our index is a consistent measure of the characteristic under investigation and not subject to fluctuations due to random error or unrelated circumstances. Validity is concerned with the questions as to whether the index is measuring what it is supposed to, and how well it does this. Validity requires reliability.

There are well recognised psychometric procedures which can be applied to determine both reliability and validity of a measure. For the assessment of reliability these include test-retest reliability, internal consistency and inter-rater reliability. Test-retest reliability is a measure of the consistency of patients responses and or scores on repeated occasions over time. The time span is chosen in order to minimise the effects of natural changes over time and can vary from days to months. Internal consistency is how well each of the items in each of the various dimensions(i.e. anxiety depression etc) correlate with one another. The logic of this is that if there are satisfactory correlations between the items within one dimension then they are all measuring the same thing. Inter-rater reliability tells how well our measure performs in the hands of different interviewers. It is an indicator of interviewer variability between interviewers with the same patient and tells us whether different interviewers record and rate similarly given the same information.

Validity can be determined in a number of ways including examination of the measures construct and predictive validity which will require the use of statistical procedures such as factor and discriminant analysis, in order to test hypotheses that the measure in fact measures what it is was designed to. Correlational studies with existing validated scales measuring psychological and physical functioning provides further supportive evidence of validity as do predictive studies in which quality of life follows disease outcome. Aspects of reliability and validity have been extensively described by Nunnally (1985), and by Kline (1986).

Problems of Measurement

Quality of life has been defined here as a multidimensional concept incorporating the affective, cognitive and social aspects of the patient's life. Subjective phenomena, such as feelings and thoughts which are representative of these aspects, are by definition unobserveable by others. Therefore, if quality of life as defined here is an unobserveable variable, its objective measurement must be via the subjective reports of the patient which are taken to be representative of the expression of the patient's quality of life.

The objective measurement of subjective judgements of the patient can be made by various procedures. The most common of these being the structured or semi structured interview and self administered questionnaire or self-report. Both approaches have their advantages and disadvantages. Interviews can be more flexible, they enable probing to find what the respondent is actually meaning, overcome the problem of reading difficulties. They also allow a rapport to develop between the interviewee and interviewer and can provide a richer source of data to be obtained. Disadvantages of interviews are that they can be costly in both time and money. Their use more often than not will be limited to those with special knowledge and interviewing skills. Questionnaires on the other hand are cheap and easy to administer. However they require a level of literacy from the respondent and extensive design and development work in wording. Despite their extensive use in the quantification of subjective data, questionnaires and interviews are subject to a number of measurement errors which effect the reliability and subsequently the validity of the measure (Meadows and Wise, 1988).

Two major sources of systematic error as opposed to random error which apply equally to both the interview and self-completion process is the response style of the patient in answering the questions. One such style which has been described as 'acquiescence' or 'yea saying', is the tendency of the respondent to answer yes or to agree to statements irrespective of their content, particularly when the statements are in the form of plausible generalities (Oppenheim 1968). Another source of systematic error which has been identified is "social desirability" which is the tendency of the respondent to agree to statements which are believed to reflect socially desirable attitudes or behaviour. Naess (1987) suggests 'idealisation' as a further response style pertinent to the measurement of quality of life and suggests idealisation may be a life style, a form...

> "of wishful thinking or defence against the harsher aspects of life"...One tells not only the surrounding world, but also oneself, that one is in very fine fettle or that everything is now going so much better.

A significant source of unreliability in the interview is interviewer variability in approach and level of rapport or failure to adhere to the interview format. Other factors known to influence the interviewer's ability to rate accurately are the generosity or leniency error, a general unwillingness to be critical or damning of others, and the halo effect which is when the rater forms an overall impression of the individual which then influences judgement on specific qualities rated.

Some Available Measures

Despite the methodological problems in the design and development of quality of life measures, a number of scales have been developed in an attempt to measure the concept.

An instrument developed for the Diabetes Control and Complications Trial (DCCT) which is an ongoing US randomised trial of two insulin treatment regimens, is the "Diabetes Quality-of-Life" measure (DQOL), (DCCT, 1988). This is a self-completion 46 core item instrument reported to measure 4 primary domains: Satisfaction, Impact, Diabetes worry and Social/Vocational worry rated on a 5 point Likert type scale. The content is non specific to forms of treatment or self monitoring. Psychometrically the instrument has shown to have both satisfactory test-retest reliability and internal consistency together with reasonable convergent validity with a number of existing validated instruments. However, the development of the instrument appears to have been done without the necessary scaling procedures and as a result there is no psychometric evidence in support of the conceptual basis of the individual domains. Furthermore a number of items appear to be age and culture specific. Clearly without further evidence in support of the psychometric qualities required of it the utility of the DQOL remains equivocal.

In Scandinavia, Hornquist (1982, 1989) has developed a quality of life package which comprises 5 self-rated life domains (somatic, psychological, social, behavioural, material and structural). Complementary to the life domain rating is the well-being rating which addresses 14 different kinds of emotions or perceptions in more detail. The content is both illness related and general. The package has been used in a number of different populations including alcohol abusers and the unemployed (Hornquist, 1989) and has shown evidence of both reliability and validity. The package has also been used in a quality of life study of adult insulin dependent patients who changed from syringe to pen injector (Hornquist et al., 1990). Reported inprovements in quality of life however referred to retrospective changes occurring as a consequence of the insulin pen. In a Norwegian study of insulin dependent patients, Hanestad (1990) reported an association between self-reported compliance and ratings on the psychological and behavioural domains of the package.

One disadvantage of the package, as Hornquist has pointed out, is that it remains unstandardised. A further consideration is that the package has been developed for use in Scandinavia, therefore prior to use in an English speaking setting it will require translation and subsequent piloting.

Scales developed by Bradley and Lewis (1990) to measure Psychological

Well-being of patients with diabetes treated with oral hypoglycaemic agents comprises 6 depression, 6 anxiety and 6 positive well-being statements. The depression and anxiety statements were selected from existing measures because they appear to be less confounded by somatic symptoms often associated with diabetic symptomatology. Each statement is self-rated on a four point Likert type scale. All 18 statements are general rather than diabetes specific. Factor analysis of the responses of 178 tablet treated patients has provided supportive evidence of the construct validity of the scale by confirming the hypothesised structure of the subscales. The internal consistency of each of the three subscales has been shown to be satisfactory for 6 item scales. A similar scale is being developed for insulin users as part of a World Health Organisation multicentre study of continuous subcutaneous insulin infusion pumps. Unpublished research has supported the structure of the subscales.

An advantage of the scales is the small number of statements and their brevity (e.g. I feel nervous and anxious). However although the scales are sufficiently general for use with healthy populations thus enabling comparability of psychological well-being of patients with diabetes with healthy populations or patients with other chronic illnesses, they are not designed to measure psychological well-being specifically attributable to diabetes. However, the psychometric properties and confirmation of the structure of the scales suggests that these measures might be a promising development in the measurement of well-being particularly when used in conjunction with more diabetes specific instruments. One such instrument is the Diabetes Health Profile currently being developed at Charing Cross Hospital (Meadows et al., 1989).

Summary and Conclusions

The measurement of quality of life in general is aimed at expanding our understanding of the thoughts, feelings and behaviour of people in order to identify what changes have to be made if one wants to improve the quality of life of the individual.

Within the context of chronic disease such as diabetes, it is now generally accepted that patho-physiological responses to illness and its treatment are not always the most appropriate means of evaluating functional outcome for the patient and attention is now directed to the assessment of quality of life.

Quality of life can be viewed as a global concept, encompassing a number of key dimensions including, psychological state, role functioning social interaction and physical status, each of which should be specific to the disease and characteristics of the patients under study.

In the construction and development of quality of life measures a number of procedural steps must be taken in order to produce a valuable and acceptable measure. Among these steps are included the processes of validity and reliability assessment. Because research strategies differ between clinical medicine and the psychosocial, a number of these steps are likely to represent a new approach for some. It is therefore important that all those involved in the development of appropriate measures of quality of life understand and accept the need for each of these procedures.

In attempting to measure the patient's quality of life, we are treading new ground. However as Schipper (1983) points out, quality of life studies ...

> will force us to come out of the comfort of technologic medicine into a world that is less concrete and less controllable but more human.

References

Bradley, C. and Lewis, K.S. (1990). Measurement of psychological well-being and Treatment Satisfaction developed from the responses of people with tablet treated diabetes. *Diabetic Medicine* 7, 445–451.

Cohen, S. and Wills, T.A. (1985). Stress, Social Support and the Buffering Hypothesis. *Psychological Bulletin* 98, 310–357.

Diabetes Control and Complications Trial Research Group (1988). Reliability and Validity of a Diabetes quality of life measure for the diabetes control and complications trial (D.C.C.T.) *Diabetes Care* 11, 725–732.

Diener, E., Emmons, A., Larsen, R.J. and Griffin, S. (1985). The satisfaction with life scale: A measure of life satisfaction. *Journal of Personality Assessment* 49, 71–75.

Ferrell, B.R., Wisdom, C. and Wenzl, C. (1989). Quality of Life as an Outcome Variable in the Management of Cancer Pain. *Cancer* 63, 2321–2327.

Ganster, C.D. and Victor, B. (1988). The impact of social support on mental and physical health. *British Journal of Medical Psychology* 61, 17–36.

Guyatt, G.H., Bombardier, C. and Tugwell, P. (1986). Measuring disease-specific quality of life in clinical trials. *Canadian Medical Association Journal.* 134, 889–895.

Hanestad, B.R. (1990). Self-assessed compliance and quality of life. *Diabetic Medicine* Supp. 1 to Vol. 7, 52.

Hornquist, J.O. (1982). The Concept of Quality of Life. *Scandinavian Journal of Social Medicine.* 10, 57–61.

Hornquist, J.O. (1989). Quality of Life: Concept and Assessment. *Scandinavian Journal of Social Medicine.* 18, 69–79.

Hornquist, J.O., Wikby, A., Andersson, P.E. and Dufva A.M. (1990). Insulin pen treatment quality of life and metabolic control: Retrospective intra-group evaluations. *Diabetes Research and Clinical Practice* (in press).

Kline, P. (1986). *A handbook of test construction.* Methuen, London.

Lewis, K.S., Bradley, C., Knight, G., Boulton, A.J.M. and Ward, J.D. (1988). A Measure of Treatment Satisfaction Designed Specifically for People with Insulin-dependent Diabetes. *Diabetic Medicine* 5, 235–242.

Liang, J. (1984). Dimensions of the Life Satisfaction Index A: A structural formulation. *Journal of Gerontology* 39, 613–622.

Meadows, K.A. and Wise, P.H. (1988). Questionnaire Design in Diabetes Care and Research No. 2: Making the Choice. *Diabetic Medicine* 5, 823–829.

Meadows, K.A., Brown, K.G., Thompson, C and Wise, P.H. (1989). The diabetes Health Questionnaire (DHQ): Preliminary validation of a new instrument. *Diabetic*

Medicine Supp. 2 to Vol. 6, **78**.

Naess, S. (1987). *Quality of life research. Concepts, methods and applications.* Institute of Applied Social Research, Oslo.

Neugarten, B.L., Havighurst, R.J. and Tobin, S. (1961). The measurement of life satisfaction. *Journal of Gerontology* **16**, 134–143.

Nunnally, J.C. (1985). *Psychometric Theory* 2nd Ed. Tata McGraw-Hill Publishing Company Limited, New Delhi.

Oppenheim, A.N. (1968). *Questionnaire design and attitude measurement.* Heinemann Educational Books Ltd.

Schafer, L.C., McCaul, K.D. and Glasgow, R.E. (1986). Supportive and Non-supportive Family Behaviours: Relationships to Adherence and Metabolic Control in Persons with Type 1 Diabetes. *Diabetes Care* **9**, 179–185.

Schipper, H. (1983). Why measure quality of life? *Canadian Medical Association Journal.* **128**, 1367–1370.

Spitzer, W.O., Dobson A.J., Hall, J. (1981). The QL-index. *Journal of Chronic Diseases.* **34**, 585–597.

Ware, J.E. (1984). Conceptualising Disease Impact and Treatment Outcomes. *Cancer* **53** (10 Supp.), 2316–2326.

Wenger, N.K. (1986). Quality of life: concept and approach to measurement. *Advances in Cardiology* **33**, 122–130.

The Economics of Diabetes Care

John Brazier and Richard Jeavons

Medical Care Research Unit, Department of Public Health Medicine, Medical School, University of Sheffield S10 2RX and the Northern General Hospital, Sheffield S5 7AU, UK.

Introduction

Economists, as purveyors of the "dismal science" of economics, inhabit a world dominated by the gloomy problem of scarcity of resources. Economics as a discipline is founded on the observation that choices in the use of resources must be made because the resources available are limited and our potential demands on the use of those resources are unlimited. From this arises the concept of "opportunity cost" *ie.* a decision to use resources to satisfy a particular demand must involve sacrificing the opportunity of obtaining the benefits of using the same resources to satisfy other demands.

Once these economic facts of life have been acknowledged, the importance of economic analysis and techniques in decision making can be appreciated. As individuals we are all involved in deciding what to purchase with our limited budgets and how to spend our time. "Efficiency" is achieved by decisions leading to a use of scarce resources which maximises benefits. In the context of health and social care in the United Kingdom, a growing body of literature on economic evaluation seeks to address the issue of how best to use the scarce (largely) public funds available to meet the health needs of the population. It attempts to tackle questions such as which technologies or treatments should be used to treat specific health problems? Which health problems should be treated and at what level? How much of the nation's resources should be devoted to health care? All these issues involve problems of choice in the use of resources and are appropriately, though not exclusively, the subject matter of economics.

Economic Evaluation

Economic evaluation has been developed by economists to assess the impact of alternative courses of action on society in terms of costs and benefits. This cost-benefit approach has been developed to assist public sector decision makers allocate scarce resources (Sugden and Williams, 1978; Mishan, 1975; and Dasgupta and Pearce, 1972). It has been applied to many areas of health care, including end stage renal disease, heart transplantation, general surgical techniques (eg. hernia repair), and drug regimes. (For reviews of studies in health care economic evaluation see Drummond, 1981 and Drummond *et al.*, 1986.) Despite a rapid growth in research activity only a minority of treatments have been subject to economic evaluation, and very little has been done on the technology of diabetes care. Here we describe the key features and difficulties with economic evaluation, and how it might be applied to diabetes care, rather than attempt a formal review of very scant literature.

The cost-benefit approach is not confined to examining the financial consequences of alternative courses of action but all types of costs and benefits (Drummond, 1980 and Drummond *et al.*, 1987). There are often many non-pecuniary costs, as well as benefits, such as time lost, discomfort and even risk of death (eg. for surgical procedures). Gerard *et al.* (1989) found the total social costs of diabetes mellitus in England and Wales in 1984 to be up to £602 m, and only 40% of this total were direct NHS costs, the rest being made up of loss in output from reduced time at work, the value of lost leisure time and so forth. The majority of benefits deriving from health care are also non-pecuniary. In the case of improved diabetes control, this would include fewer hospitalisations for various complications, and improved mobility and visual acuity which enable a person to continue contributing to the Gross National Product. But no-one, least of all an economist, would wish to measure the value of health care, only in terms of its ability to maintain people as productive members of the workforce. The most important benefit of health care, as its name suggests, is likely to be the person's well being associated with improved health status.

There are enormous difficulties in measuring and valuing non pecuniary costs and benefits, but this does not mean they can be ignored. Health service decisions determined solely on the grounds of accountancy are likely to be misinformed. Valuing non pecuniary costs and benefits can not be avoided. For example, the decision to fund a kidney dialysis programme which costs £18,000 a year for each patient, implies that the value placed on a kidney patient's life is at least equal to or more than £18,000. By the same deduction, a decision not to fund such a programme (nor any alternative way of saving these patients lives) implies a value less than the cost. These implicit valuations are being made by individuals, medical practitioners and other providers, and health authorities on behalf of the NHS and hence society. Typically, decisions are being made in ignorance of all the costs and benefits of the treatments, and hence significant variation has been found in the implied value attached to the same health benefit in different contexts (Mooney, 1977). For example, policies pursued to avoid repetition of the Ronan Point disaster, when a large block of flats collapsed, have been estimated to imply a value of approximately £20,000,000 per life saved. As an investment of scarce resources in saving life this gave a poor return compared to kidney dialysis or even heart transplantation (Drummond, 1980, Williams, 1985).

While its principles may be simple, economic evaluation is not objective, since it necessarily contains subjective valuations of costs and benefits. What it does is make any value judgments explicit. This process begins with the identification of benefits (such as extended life, reduced disability, better eyesight and so on), their measurement and finally their valuation. The first, and probably most important question is whose values to use – the patient, the medical practitioner or society as a whole? In a social cost benefit analysis economists tend to adopt a societal perspective, and so attempt to use the values of all. There are other ethical positions, for example to only use the values of taxpayers. Inevitably, this issue is a source of conflict but the economist is only interested in being clear as to who's values are being used. A typical example would be in the evaluation of care for the elderly infirm where the costs and benefits to the elderly person must be balanced with those to their family as informal carers. Similar issues will arise in the context of diabetes where the individual's behaviour in managing their diabetes can have knock on costs and benefits for their family and friends.

Conceptually the most powerful technique in economic evaluation is cost benefit analysis (CBA), since all costs and benefits are valued in money terms. The choice of money as a unit of account enables all effects to be compared using a single numeraire (in theory other units of account could be used, one oceanic society chooses to use rare seashells). The key problem is how to value the benefits of a health care programme in improving the quality and duration of life. In a market, an individual's valuations are reflected in their willingness to pay for health gains, such as improved life-expectancy. One example are the compensating wage differentials for workers in risky occupations (Jones – Lee, et al., 1985). In health care, market values alone are regarded as inadequate measures of society's values (see later for an explanation). Economists have therefore either attempted to adjust market values for these imperfections, or conducted "willingness to pay" experiments where individuals are asked what they would be willing to pay for a specified health improvement (Drummond, 1980). The main criticisms of this approach are the hypothetical nature of the question, and that responses will depend in part on existing income distributions, which the NHS may wish to ignore (eg. it could lead to the 'diseases of affluence' receiving a higher weighting because of the higher incomes of sufferers).

Health economists have sought to overcome these measurement problems by addressing what are regarded as lower level efficiency questions. This means, instead of attempting to answer the question of whether an action is worthwhile, economic evaluation lowers its sights, and considers whether a particular action is the best means of achieving a given objective. The technique for doing this is cost-effectiveness analysis (CEA) which compares the costs of an action with its effects measured in 'natural' or unvalued units such as lives saved or blood glucose control. This approach is not to be confused with 'disease costing' which only estimates the total social *cost* of a disease (eg. Gerard *et al.,* 1989; and Laing and Williams, 1989) and not the effects of actions to prevent or treat it. Merely because diabetes costs society around half a billion pounds per year does not imply resources should be allocated to diabetes programmes. Determining priorities for diabetes care requires information on the cost and benefit effects of altering the level of different care programmes. For example, a study question could be whether a shared care model of care, versus a centralised hospital service, is less costly at achieving blood glucose control, or achieves improved control at a given cost. What CEA is unable to do is to assess whether achieving a particular objective, such as controlling blood glucose, is worthwhile *per se*. Health economists therefore prefer to choose an objective which is as close as possible to final outcome, such as reduced disability or improved visual acuity.

The main problem with CEA is that health care benefits are usually multi-dimensional. Problems arise, for example, where a medical intervention on the one hand results in a health improvement for most patients, but for a few there is a risk of mortality (eg. hysterectomy). The question is how to trade one health change for another. An important development aimed at address-ing this problem has been cost utility analysis (CUA) which places all health effects on one dimension – the quality adjusted life year (QALY). This allows the value of alternative health care programmes to be compared within a health services budget. In the UK this approach has been applied by researchers based at the University of York. The York method uses a 29 state classification of health with two dimensions, disability and distress (Williams, 1985). In the original study 70 respondents were asked to place a value between zero and one for each health state, where these values are the end points of death and perfect health respectively. The results from this initial study are very crude, and there is a major research programme to develop the methodology. The critical literature on QALYs has been growing rapidly (eg. Ashmore *et al.*, 1989; Carr-Hill, 1989; and Appleby and Loomes, 1987), and considerable research and testing has yet to be done in order to address questions of validity. Alternative methods of measuring QALYs have been developed by Torrance and others at McMaster University in Canada, which use expected utility theory (Torrance, 1986).

Different technologies and programmes aimed at diabetes will involve costs and benefits over different time spans which must be compared on a consistent basis to support decisions about the use of scarce resources. Many of the benefits of care for people with diabetes, particularly Type II, are long term. The temptation for decision makers with scarce resources at their disposal is to give priority to services for short term emergencies such as diabetic ketoacidosis rather than to the less immediate risks of Type II diabetes. An economic evaluation would persuade against taking such a short term view by placing a value on all costs and benefits whenever they fall. However this would not mean placing the same value on costs or benefits which occur at different times because society is not indifferent about when it bears costs and receives benefits.

In general society prefers to delay bearing costs for as long as possible and to receive benefits as soon as possible. Evidence of this "time preference" is seen clearly in the positive rate of interest we pay for borrowing money and expect to receive for lending money. Many people are prepared to pay more overall for a car by buying it on hire purchase in order to drive it now. This preference extends to health care but it is less clear by how much society prefers good health or saving lives now to good health or saving lives next year, in ten years or even fifty years time (Sugden and Williams, 1978). Economists in the United Kingdom have usually adopted a time preference rate of 6% per annum in line with the Treasury's guidance for public investment decisions.

Having used economic evaluation to compare alternative health care programmes for a group such as those with diabetes, a common mistake is to presume that the results are universally applicable, disregarding differences between individuals and their existing circumstances. In practice a decision maker is not usually concerned with all or nothing but options for incremental expansion or contraction of different programmes aimed at different target groups. A district health authority may be considering an additional outpatient session for the consultant with special interest in diabetes, a community based "walk in" education centre, the extension of shared care and setting up of a register or a change in screening protocols. Each of these options is relatively small compared to the total service for diabetes and a decision maker needs to understand what differential effects or benefits they may bring depending on the age, type and severity of illness, and social background of the target population. Economists refer to the marginal costs and benefits of a programme when discussing the evaluation of these types of changes to service provision. In principle the ultimate margin would be a change in treatment for an individual patient but in practice formal economic evaluation concentrates on groups of patients and, therefore, more significant resource allocation problems. On this basis there is clear scope for a conflict of interest between an assessment of an individual's needs, as defined by clinical judgment and pursued through clinical freedom, and the needs of a target population as defined by a policy on service provision informed by evaluation of the alternatives.

Economic evaluation is a developing field which has many methodological and practical problems. Critics have been concerned that, given these problems, economic evaluation should not be used to make decisions (Klein, 1989). Economists would agree with this view and have argued that economic evaluation can only ever be an aid to decision making since value judgments play a major role in its practical application. In addition decision makers have to consider objectives other than efficiency such as notions of equity, choice, and political pressures. Economic evaluation is a framework for systematically examining the costs and benefits of options and explicitly taking account of the necessary value judgments, as well as technical judgments, in choosing between them. This approach would seem particularly relevant to the expanding area of the technology of diabetes care, with the large array of alternative means to help people with diabetes achieve a better life.

Homo Economicus with Diabetes

Economic evaluation should be used in the evaluation of alternative approaches to diabetes care to aid policy decisions on what services to provide. Economics as a discipline also has a contribution to make in our attempts to understand the behaviour of individuals with diabetes towards their condition and diabetes care. In traditional consumer theory the principles of weighing up costs and benefits in decisions about the use of scarce resources are applied to the individual's behaviour. Individuals are predicted to choose their purchases of goods and services to maximise their utility or happiness, on the basis of the following:

1. Their wants or tastes which reflect the relative value of the benefit they derive from different goods and services.
2. Their choice set or resources in terms of income, time and so on.
3. The costs of goods and services in financial terms (price) and less tangible dimensions such as time, inconvenience and discomfort.

In this model of individual behaviour a person with diabetes would compare the costs and benefits of diabetes care (e.g. time and money spent monitoring blood glucose and attending clinics for better health status in ten years time) with alternatives (e.g. using the time and money to socialise with friends and have a good time) and do the things which give them most benefit for the cost incurred.

Consumer theory is also concerned with predicting the consequences of changes in choice sets and prices. Hence, for example, an increase in income or a reduction in price would *a priori* be expected to increase the demand for a 'normal' good. (There are exceptions, for a detailed exposition see Hirshleifer, 1988.) In the context of diabetes care, moving a screening clinic to a more accessible location, thereby reducing time and travel costs to the target population would, all things being equal, be expected to increase attendance rates. Introduction of a more convenient and effective method of monitoring blood glucose would be expected to increase monitoring activity. Equally, participation in any voluntary diabetes care activity might be increased by offering financial inducements which effectively reduced the costs of participation to the individual. But it is important to note that even where individuals face identical costs and have the same choice set the theory would predict differences in consumption of diabetes care by the observation that people place different values on the benefits to be derived from it. In consumer theory therefore we have a model of individual behaviour towards diabetes and diabetes care which could be tested in terms of its ability to explain observed differences in actual behaviour.

An important principle underlying this model of behaviour is that the individual is the best judge of their own interest (ie. knows the relative benefits of different goods and service) and has the right to pursue that interest in an unfettered way. Economists have shown that under certain assumptions, the problem of how to allocate scarce resources in the best interests of society can be solved by the operation of a free market in which individuals, pursuing their own self interest, trade with each other. This is the invisible hand hypothesis first put forward by Adam Smith in 'The Wealth of Nations' where he observes.

> "It is not from the benevolence of the butcher, the brewer, or the baker, that we expect our dinner, but from their regard to their own interest." (Smith, 1776).

Critics of markets have often been repulsed by the underlying motivation of greed. Economists are instrumentalists who have argued that if markets can achieve society's ends, then why should how they work matter? The pro-marketeers would therefore leave individuals to purchase diabetes care in the market place, like the more conventional textbook economic goods such as brussel sprouts and video recorders.

But to what extent does diabetes care share the characteristics of brussel sprouts in the eyes of the consumer and society?

Health economists have long recognised that the traditional model of consumer theory involves a too naive and simplistic view of the nature of health care (see for example Arrow, 1963 and Culyer, 1971) particularly in the presumption of consumer sovereignty, that individuals bear all the costs and benefits of their actions, and that they are in a position to judge the value of all costs and benefits (Mooney, 1986). The first is rarely true in the consumption of health care since the consumer is not the only recipient of any benefits, there are benefits to others from reducing the incidence of contagious diseases such as AIDS. More importantly there are also external benefits in the form of a humanitarian concern for others, as witnessed by charities such as the British Diabetic Association and indeed by the NHS itself (though even this concern could still be argued as being motivated by self interest). In the NHS, the financial costs of health care are principally borne by society as a whole and hence an individual's decision to consume health care also affects others. This divergence of individual and collective interests suggests the former acting on self interest will not necessarily act in the best interest of society.

Equally important in health care is the information available to individuals at the point of decision making. Health care is an unusual 'good' in that it is usually unpleasant, costly and in many cases dangerous. Individuals only suffer these costs in the anticipation of their impact on health. This characteristic would not be a problem in a free market but for the fact that consumers are often ignorant of the relationship between health care and health. Consumers may be the best judge of the benefits to them of a particular health state but they cannot be regarded as being the best judges of the means of obtaining health. Even *ex post* a patient may not know whether health care was responsible for any change in their (or others') health state.

Patients consult with doctors and other perceived experts partly to overcome this lack of information. What is unusual, though not unique to health care, is that the complexity of this information and the low health status of many of the patients means they often willingly transfer decision making to doctors. This is the well-known 'agency relationship'.

The 'perfect' agency relationship has been described as where a doctor makes a decision on behalf of a patient which is the same as the patient would have made faced with the same technical information (Culyer, 1989). This requires the doctor to subsume totally not only their own interests (e.g. to maximise income) but also to know and use the patient's own tastes such as the patient's relative valuations of different health dimensions, risk-bearing and time preference. In essence doctors are not only providers but also the effective buyers of health care on behalf of the patients who come to them for their services. This is a potential source of conflict which has been a central concern to health economists (e.g. Evans, 1984). Perhaps characteristically, economists have empirically tested this conflict by examining whether doctors behaviour is influenced by the method of remuneration (Sloan and Feldman, 1978; Pauly, 1980).

As principal financier, the Government has traditionally relied on the medical profession to prevent exploitation of the agency relationship by self-regulation. The profession has long claimed they are ethically bound to offer the most beneficial treatment to their patient (with its classic expression in the Hippocratic oath), and by implication, regardless of cost. In a cash limited environment more care for one group of patients means less for another group. Despite the rhetoric, in practice clinicians have never been able to fulfill their supposed ethical obligation to all patients due to resource constraints set by their hospital, health authority and ultimately Government. Economists' main concern has been that clinicians should become more aware of the costs and benefits of different actions and use these in combination to guide their decisions.

The roles of hospitals, health authorities and Government as other agents in the process of determining resource allocation in health care have been clarified and reinforced as part of the National Health Service reforms. Health authorities and budget holding general practitioners will set priorities for health care within a broad policy framework provided by Government, by taking the role of purchaser on behalf of their catchment population in a contract negotiation with providers of services. It is to be assumed that in playing this role, their main objective will be to purchase that health care which will maximise the health status of the population.

The derivation of the demand for health care, such as technology of diabetes care, is therefore the result of a complex series of decisions by three different actors – the individual with diabetes, the doctor (or other 'experts') and the purchasing agency (e.g. health authority). These three agents can be incorporated into the conventional economic model, with each making decisions to maximise their objectives within the constraints of their choice set. The roles of the agents in determining the final allocations of resources to diabetes care are set out in figure 1. Individuals with undiagnosed diabetes may experience symptoms such as weight loss, thirst and daytime tiredness leading to a 'want' for better health. They then decide whether to convert 'wants' into 'demand' for medical help by weighing up the costs of a consultation (time, travel, a fee, the fear of finding our something they did not want to know) and benefits (potential gains in health status). The medical practitioner makes a diagnosis and assesses the need for treatment. Clearly many needs will not be seen and many demands may be assessed as not in need of treatment. Resources must then be rationed between competing needs, including diabetes care, by medical practitioners and health authorities. For example, a GP refers the patient to a hospital specialist, who in turn decides the patient's 'need' to attend a diabetes centre. However, the health authority regards such a centre as a low priority, does not fund it, and so the patient attends outpatient clinics for treatment. In diabetes care particularly, an important final stage is where the individual distributes scarce personal resources between competing wants, and decides on the quantity and mix of available diabetes care to consume. This is referred to by practitioners as 'patient compliance'.

Figure 1 *The derivation of the demand for diabetes care (after Cooper, 1975)*

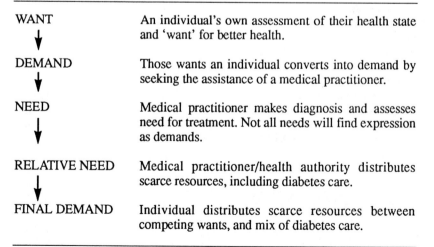

WANT	An individual's own assessment of their health state and 'want' for better health.
DEMAND	Those wants an individual converts into demand by seeking the assistance of a medical practitioner.
NEED	Medical practitioner makes diagnosis and assesses need for treatment. Not all needs will find expression as demands.
RELATIVE NEED	Medical practitioner/health authority distributes scarce resources, including diabetes care.
FINAL DEMAND	Individual distributes scarce resources between competing wants, and mix of diabetes care.

Understanding the demand for health care is important for implementing the findings of economic evaluation. If it is found that the benefits to society of controlling blood glucose levels in people with Type II diabetes in terms of improved GNP, reduced NHS costs, and the enhanced health of recipients outweighs the costs, then steps must be taken to ensure this policy is translated into demand. Society can intervene to increase individual demand for initial medical assistance by reducing costs, such as travel time, and improving perceived benefit by providing better information on the effects of treatment. Similarly compliance with a recommended dietary regimen can be influenced by providing more convenient support and advice. More controversially, the economist's model would predict individual behaviour could be influenced by more direct incentives to seek and comply with treatments, such as offering a payment to those who control their blood glucose. It has also been suggested that ill health which results from knowing neglect of health through life style habits such as smoking or a failure to comply with treatments should not be dealt with free by the NHS. This position would suggest such people should pay for the consequences of poor blood glucose control. This punitive approach raises complex technical questions of how to prove a particular illness, such as end stage renal disease actually resulted from poor blood glucose control, and profound ethical questions. Currently the position implied through NHS provision is that individuals should not be discriminated against in this way.

Another way of altering the demand for a good such as diabetes care is to change people's taste or preference for it. Conventionally, economics assumes peoples tastes are given, and it has no interest in how they were formed. This may seem a naive assumption, but it is simply intended to set a boundary around the discipline of economics. This is a point at which other social science disciplines are more willing to take up the intellectual challenge and the formation of people's tastes for health is something which psychologists and sociologists have studied, though couched in different terms. The extent to which society should attempt to alter peoples tastes by applying such knowledge is more controversial, and is also an ethical matter. Some believe people's tastes are in some sense sacrosanct, while others argue that society's interests should dominate. This is a time honoured debate which should be conducted explicitly, rather than resolved implicitly by the actions of health professionals.

Summary and Conclusions

Economics, with its all pervading subject matter of the scarcity of resources, should be a significant contributor to a greater understanding of the technology of diabetes care and the process of bringing diabetes care to those with diabetes. Despite its methodological and practical problems, economic evaluation is a framework which should be part of every evaluation, since it ensures that both the costs and benefits of alternatives are considered. Perhaps most importantly, it knows its own limitations as a decision aiding technique and makes the necessary value judgments in decision making more explicit. In doing so, it forces us to consider ethical questions about whose values count, the interdependence of individuals' well being and the potential conflict between individual and collective interest.

In consumer theory, economics offers a model of individual behaviour which may provide some insight into patients' compliance with recommended treatments and the roles of other agents in the delivery of diabetes care. Within this model, the costs of diabetes care and the choice set of the person with diabetes may be varied (through explicit policies) but their tastes or values associated with the benefits of diabetes care are regarded as innate and unalterable. The underlying assumption remains that the individual is the best judge of their own interest and that society is best served by allowing individuals to pursue their own interests. In this context, diabetes education must be seen as ensuring that people with diabetes are fully informed of the consequences of their actions rather than as a means of changing their values.

The application of economics to the technology of diabetes care suggests the need for working interfaces with three other broad disciplines. Firstly and most obviously, with the clinicians providing diabetes care so that a full understanding of the technology and its effectiveness is gained. This interface has been developing over recent years into a better mutual understanding of perspective and approach. Secondly, economics has a long tradition of an active interface with moral philosophy and ethics which should not be ignored or forgotten in the application of economic principles to the problem of allocating resources for health care. Diabetes care is one area where ethical issues raised by conflicts between individual and collective interests are particularly prominent. Finally, economics offers a simple model of human behaviour which leaves the door wide open for more sophisticated approaches involving other behavioural sciences. It is perhaps this final interface which requires the most effort if it is to be defined more clearly and useful collaborative work promoted.

References

Appleby, L. and Loomes, G. (1987). The validity of QALYs for Medical decsion making. Paper presented to the Health Economics Study Group, June 1987.

Arrow, K.J. (1963). Uncertainty and the welfare economics of medical care. *The American Economic Review*, 53, 941–73.

Ashmore, M., Mulkay, M. and Pinch, T. (1989). *Health and Efficiency: a Sociology of Health Economics*. Milton Keynes: Open University Press.

Carr-Hill, R.A. (1989). Assumptions of the QALY Procedure. *Social Science and Medicine*, 29, 469–77.

Cooper, M.H. (1975). *Rationing Health Care*. London: Croom Helm.

Culyer, A.J. (1971). The Nature of the Commodity 'Health Care' and its efficient allocation. *Oxford Economic Papers*, **23**, 189–211.

Culyer, A.J. (1989). The normative economics of health care finance and provision. *Oxford Review of Economic Policy*, **5**, 1:34–58.

Dasgupta, A.K. and Pearce, D.W. (1972). *Cost-benefit analysis: theory and practice.* London: MacMillan.

Drummond, M.F. (1980). *Principles of Economic Appraisal in Health Care.* Oxford: Oxford University Press.

Drummond, M.F. (1981). *Studies in economic appraisal in health care.* Oxford: Oxford University Press.

Drummond, M.F., Ludbrook, A., Lowson, K.V. and Steele, A. (1986). *Studies in economic appraisal in health care, vol 2.* Oxford: Oxford University Press.

Drummond, M.F., Stoddart, G.E. and Torrance, G.W. (1987). *Methods of economic evaluation of health care programme.* Oxford: Oxford Medical Publications, 338.473621.

Evans, R.G. (1984). *Strained Mercy: The Economics of Canadian Health Care.* Butterworth: Toronto.

Gerard, K., Donaldson, C. and Maynard, A.K. (1989). The Cost of Diabetes. *Diabetic Medicine*, **6**, 164–170.

Hirshleifer, J. (1988). *Price Theory and Applications. 4th Edition.* London: Prentice – Hall International (UK) Editions.

Jones-Lee, M.W., Hammerton, M. and Philips, P.R. (1985). 'The Value of Safety: results of a national sample survey'. *The Economic Journal*, **95**, pp. 49–72.

Klein, R. (1989). The role of health economics: Rosencrantz to medicine's Hamlet. *British Medical Journal*, **229**, 275–76.

Laing, W. and Williams, R. (1989). *Diabetes: A model of health care management.* London: Office of Health Economics.

Mishan, E.J. (1975). *Cost-benefit analysis.* London: George Allen and Unwin.

Mooney, G.H. (1977). *The Valuation of Human Life.* London: MacMillan.

Mooney, G.H. (1986). *Economics, Medicine and Health Care.* Brighton: Wheatsheaf books.

Pauly, M.V. (1980). *Doctors and Their Workshops.* Chicago: University of Chicago press.

Sloan, F.A. and Feldman, R. (1978). Competition Among Physicians in Greenberg, W. (ed). *Competition in the Health Care Sector: Past, Present and Future.* Germantown: Aspen Systems.

Smith, A. (1776). *An inquiry into the Nature and Causes of the Wealth of Nations.* E. Cannan (ed.), London: Methuen.

Sugden, R. and Williams, A. (1978). *The Principles of Practical Cost – benefit analysis.* Oxford: Oxford University Press.

Torrance, G.W. (1986). Measurement of health state utilities for economic appraisal. *Journal of Health Economics*, **5**, 1–30.

Williams, A. (1985). Economics of Coronary Artery Bypass Grafting. *British Medical Journal*, **291**, 326–329.

Glossary

Amperometric/amperometry

Current measurement at a constant voltage.

Analyte

A chemical substance measured by a system or device, e.g. glucose.

Behavioural Medicine

An interdisciplinary approach to the interactions between behaviour and bodily states of health and illness. The term Behavioural Medicine was first used in the early 1970's.

Biocompatibility

The ability of a material to perform adequately with an appropriate host response in a specific application. Commonly taken to be a reaction of the body to a device such as a glucose sensor, and the effects of such a reaction on the function of the device.

Biosensor

A small measuring probe incorporating a biological recognition molecule such as an enzyme or antibody.

British Diabetic Association: 10 Queen Anne Street, London, WIM 0BD, U.K.

The association formed in 1934 with the aims of supporting people living with diabetes and for research into diabetes. Membership is open to anyone.

Brittle diabetes

Diabetes which is so unstable that the patient is recurrently precipitated into high or low blood glucose levels sufficient to interrupt their daily activities and often precipitates recurrent admission to hospital.

Closed-loop systems

Systems in which there is feedback control. For example a glucose sensor can be linked to an insulin pump to produce closed-loop control of insulin delivery in diabetic patients (an 'artificial endocrine pancreas').

215

Continuous Subcutaneous Insulin Infusion (CSII) Pump

An externally worn device for delivering insulin via a cannula and needle inserted under the skin, usually of the abdomen. Insulin can be delivered continually throughout the day with booster doses delivered by pressing a button on the pump when extra insulin is required at meal times. Some CSII pumps are programmable to allow adjustment of rates of insulin delivery according to the time of day or night.

Diabetic Control and Complications Trial (DCCT)

Multicentre trial investigating the effects of tight control of blood glucose levels on the development of retinopathy and other diabetes-related complications in patients with Type 1 diabetes.

Ex vivo

Outside of the body, e.g. measurements taken in blood pumped out of the patient into a device.

Field-Effect Transistor

A micro-electronic device for measuring electrical potential.

GhB

See Glycosylated Haemoglobin.

Glucose oxidase

An enzyme catalysing the oxidation of glucose to gluconic acid and hydrogen peroxide. Obtained from microbial sources e.g. Aspergillus niger. Frequently used as the recognition molecule in glucose sensors (biosensors).

Glucose sensors

Devices for the measurement of glucose levels in blood or tissues. A sensor resides permanently in one position and by electrochemical means produces a current proportional to the glucose concentration, that current being measured externally.

Glycosylated Haemoglobin

A compound formed by combination of glucose and haemoglobin in the blood, the concentration of which is proportional to the average blood glucose concentration over the previous two months. The compound is known as haemoglobin A_1, it can be separated from ordinary haemoglobin A in the laboratory, and its concentration measured.

HbA₁

See glycosylated haemoglobin.

Health Beliefs

Beliefs about health and illness which may be held by anyone including health professionals as well as patients. The "Health Belief Model" is perhaps the best well known of the several models which attempt to show how beliefs can influence behaviour and, hence, health and illness.

Hypoglycaemia

Low blood glucose concentrations. There is no accepted definition of how low blood glucose values must be reduced for the term to be used, although most non-diabetic subjects have clear signs and symptoms of hypoglycaemia below 2.2 mmol/l (40 mg/dl).

Immunosensor

A biosensor incorporating antibody as the recognition molecule.

Implantable insulin pumps

Insulin delivery devices intended for implantation under the skin, and delivering insulin continually through a cannula into the peritoneal cavity or the great veins. These devices can be programmed from outside the body to change the insulin delivery rate, for example at meal times.

In vivo

Inside the body, e.g. an implanted glucose sensor.

In vitro

Studies or measurements performed in the laboratory, remote from the patient or subject. In vitro literally means "in glass" and often refers to measurements performed in a test tube.

Locus of Control

A term deriving from social psychology used to refer to the perceived source of control of one's behaviour. In its simplest form it is operationalised as a single dimension running from high internal control to high external control, with the highly internal individual feeling in control of outcomes while the highly external individual feels that control is unobtainable or resides elsewhere. Recent developments in conceptualising locus of control have led to multidimensional measures of locus of control where externality is subdivided into notions of 'chance' factors on the one hand controlling outcomes and 'powerful others' being in control on the other.

Mediated electron transfer

A technology for glucose sensing in which a small molecular weight mediator (e.g. ferrocene) shuttles electrons directly from an enzyme to an underlying electrode.

Nephropathy

Damage to the kidneys, in the diabetic patient usually due to diabetes. Diabetic nephropathy generally progresses slowly to complete renal failure requiring transplantation or dialysis.

Neuropathy

Damage to the peripheral nervous system (that part of the nervous system other than the brain and central nervous system) usually in the diabetic patient as a result of diabetes. Peripheral neuropathy results in damage to the long nerves from the feet, hence causing numbness in the feet and predisposing to ulceration, or producing unpleasant symptoms. Autonomic neuropathy affects nerves such as those controlling the heart, blood vessels and gut, and can result in disturbances of blood pressure control, sweating and emptying of the stomach.

Pen Injectors

A device, the size and shape of a large pen, for injecting insulin.

Potentiometry

Measurement of voltage changes.

Psychometrics

The branches of psychology concerned with the measurement of psychological phenomena including knowledge, beliefs, well-being, aptitude, intelligence and personality.

Psychosomatics

That approach to medicine which emphasises the interdependence of mind and body. It is now becoming generally recognised that it is misleading to refer to only some medical conditions as 'psychosomatic' as psychosomatic issues are, to a greater or lesser extent, involved in the onset and /or course of all illness, disease and injury.

Reliability

In psychological testing and in measurement generally, this term refers to the dependability of a measurement or test. There are many aspects of reliability and methods of determining reliability but all are concerned with *consistency;* both internal consistency and (where appropriate) consistency across time commonly known as test-retest reliability

Self-monitoring of blood glucose

Measurement by the patient him/herself of the concentration of glucose in the blood, by obtaining a small drop of blood from a finger prick, and applying it to a reagent strip for a timed period. Colour development is then read visually against a chart, or a meter. Devices are now being developed to measure glucose levels directly with a glucose sensor.

Type 1 Diabetes

Often known as insulin-dependent diabetes, this type of diabetes usually but not exclusively develops in younger people, due to destruction of the pancreatic islet B-cells, and usually proceeds to complete insulin deficiency (and therefore absolute dependence on insulin).

Type 2 Diabetes

Commonly known as non-insulin dependent diabetes, this condition normally but not exclusively arises in older people, and is associated both with extreme tissue resistance to insulin, and an inability to overcome that resistance by compensatory increase in insulin secretion. Treatment is often by diet alone, or supplemented with drugs which increase insulin secretion, but many patients require insulin by injection therapy.

Validity

In psychological testing and in measurement generally, a test is valid if it measures what it claims to measure (e.g. it has concurrent validity or construct validity) and is useful (e.g. it has predictive validity or discriminant validity).

Youth Diabetes Project

A project supported by the BDA and Novo-Nordisk (UK) for the 17–25 age group that currently includes a Youth Diabetes Conference, a course for youngsters with diabetes, a course for professionals working with this age group and a quarterly newsletter.

Index